EVERYTHING CARDIOPULMONARY GUIDE

Nourishing Recipes for Thriving with Chronic bronchitis, Chronic Obstructive Pulmonary Disease (COPD), Congestive Heart Failure, and Emphysema

Joe Miller, RD

COPYRIGHT PAGE

Copyright © 2024 Joe Miller, RD

All rights reserved. No part of this publication may be reproduced, distributed, or transmitted in any form or by any means, including photocopying, recording, or other electronic or mechanical methods, without the prior written permission of the publisher, except in the case of brief quotation embodied in critical reviews and certain other non-commercial uses permitted by copyright law.

Table of Contents

COPYRIGHT PAGE 2

Table of Contents 3

INTRODUCTION 1

BRIEF OVERVIEW OF CARDIOPULMONARY DISEASES 5

Categories of cardiopulmonary disease 8

The impact of cardiovascular disease on the absorption and utilization of nutrients. 26

DIETARY NEEDS FOR PATIENTS WITH CARDIOPULMONARY DISEASE 30

The significance of dietary interventions in managing cardiopulmonary diseases. 34

Describing the distinctive nutritional needs of individuals afflicted with cardiopulmonary ailments. 38

FOODS TO AVOID IF YOU HAVE CARDIOPULMONARY DISEASE 43

    The way specific foods can worsen symptoms or increase the likelihood of complications........... 47

FOODS TO INCLUDE IN A DIET FOR CARDIOVASCULAR DISEASE 51

    Ways in which these food items can mitigate symptoms and reduce risk factors. 56

CARDIOPULMONARY DIET RECIPES 59

BREAKFAST 59

    Hearty Raspberry Pancakes 59

    Hearty Almond Pancakes 61

    Hearty Oatmeal Bread 62

    Hearty Baked Oatmeal 64

    Hearty Quiche 67

    Heart-Healthy Vanilla Blueberry Muffins 69

    Heart Healthy Breakfast: Avocado Toast 70

Seitan Burritos 72

Strawberry Rosemary Mojito 74

Balsamic Fried Eggs 76

Cranberry Ginger Almond Crunch Muffins ... 78

Basil Goat Cheese Toast with Fresh Peaches .. 80

Banana, Blueberry, and Pecan Pancakes 81

Soft-Scrambled Eggs "Alla Gricia" 84

Day- After Casserole for a Hearty Breakfast ... 86

LUNCH AND DINNER 89

Simple Seasoned Adzuki Beans 89

Hearty Spicy Kale and Pork Soup / Stew with White Beans 92

Hearty Hamburger Helper with Wagyu Beef. 94

Matelote (Fish Stew) 97

The Ultimate Hearty Minestrone 102

Hearty Tortellini and Spinach Soup 105

Sweet Corn Butter From Whitney Wright..... 107

Welsh Cawl 109

The Cuban 112

Zurek (Polish Hangover Soup) 118

Italian Wedding Soup With Parm Broth........ 123

Quinoa & Roasted Sweet Potato Superfood Salad 127

Oma's Chicken Paprikash 129

DESSERTS 132

Pudding & Custard 132

Pears En Pillowette with Almond Mascarpone Cream 134

Tang Yuan (Glutinous Rice Balls) 138

Raspberry-Lime Parfaits with Whipped Goat Cheese 142

Huckleberry Yogurt Pseudo Trifle 144

Darjeeling Tea Pain Perdu with Condensed Milk Butter 145

Chili Chocolate Mousse Cake 148

Pumpkin Pots de Creme with Orange Cranberry Whipped Cream 151

Dark Chocolate Bark 154

Roasted Peaches and Yogurt 155

Intense Strawberry Coconut Ice Cream + Almond Waffle Cone 158

No-Bake Berries & Cream Cake 162

Gingerbread Porter Cake with Cacao Nibs ... 165

SNACKS 172

Balilah with Preserved Lemons and Pomegranates 172

Bar Pizza-It's What You Crave 174

Broccoli Rabe & Fresh Mozzarella Panini 176

Roman Zucchini Fritters with Parmigiano Cheese 180

Potato, Mushroom & Caramelized Onion Pierogi 183

Basil Goat Cheese Toast with Fresh Peaches 189

Creamy Soup of Hearty Nuts, Apple, Celery Root and Sage 190

Easiest, Cheesiest Skillet Dip 193

Artichoke & potato tarte................................... 196

SUMMATION... 202

INTRODUCTION

Cardiopulmonary disease, a term encompassing a spectrum of serious health conditions affecting the heart and lungs, underscores the intricate connection between these vital organs. When one encounters trouble, it often reverberates to affect the other. For instance, if the heart struggles to efficiently pump blood, it disrupts the normal flow of oxygen in the lungs, resulting in symptoms like shortness of breath. Conversely, lung issues can force the heart to labor harder to oxygenate the blood adequately.

Heart disease holds a grim distinction as the primary cause of mortality globally, claiming the lives of over 800,000 Americans annually, without regard for gender or race. This staggering statistic translates to one in every four deaths or, in stark terms, one life lost every 36 seconds. The World Health Organization's mortality rankings starkly highlight stroke and chronic obstructive pulmonary disease (COPD) as close contenders following heart disease. Interestingly, this trend seems to intensify in nations with higher GDPs, prompting a critical examination of why preventable cardiopulmonary conditions exact such a heavy toll in first-world countries.

Yet, amidst these grim statistics, lies a beacon of hope in understanding and combating cardiopulmonary diseases. Education, prevention, and early intervention play pivotal roles in mitigating their impact. By raising awareness about risk factors such as smoking, poor diet, sedentary lifestyle, and genetic predispositions, individuals can take proactive steps to safeguard their heart and lung health. Moreover, advancements in medical research and technology offer promising avenues for early detection, personalized treatment plans, and innovative interventions aimed at improving outcomes for those affected by cardiopulmonary diseases.

While cardiopulmonary diseases cast a formidable shadow over global health, they also serve as a rallying point for concerted efforts in research, prevention, and treatment. By fostering collaboration among healthcare professionals, policymakers, researchers, and the public, we can strive to reduce the burden of cardiopulmonary diseases and pave the way toward a healthier future for generations to come.

Everything Cardiopulmonary Guide 4

CHAPTER 1
BRIEF OVERVIEW OF CARDIOPULMONARY DISEASES

Cardiopulmonary diseases encompass a spectrum of conditions affecting both the heart and lungs, often interlinked due to the intricate anatomical and functional relationship between these vital organs. The impact of these conditions, ranging from mild inconveniences to severe debilitation, can profoundly influence individuals' quality of life. Let's delve into some prevalent cardiovascular diseases:

1. Coronary artery disease manifests as the narrowing or blockage of these crucial blood vessels, leading to diminished blood flow and, in severe cases, precipitating heart attacks.

2. Heart failure presents symptoms such as fatigue, shortness of breath, and fluid retention, arising from the heart's inability to adequately pump blood to meet the body's demands.

3. Pulmonary hypertension, a subtype of hypertension, involves the constriction of pulmonary arteries, imposing greater resistance to blood flow from the heart to the lungs.

4. Chronic obstructive pulmonary disease (COPD) encompasses a cluster of lung ailments characterized by breathing difficulties and compromised lung function, including emphysema and chronic bronchitis.

5. Asthma exacerbates breathing difficulties as inflamed and constricted airways impede the flow of air in and out of the lungs.

6. Pulmonary fibrosis entails the thickening and scarring of lung tissue, impairing lung function and diminishing respiratory capacity.

Addressing symptoms and averting complications associated with these cardiopulmonary diseases typically necessitates a multifaceted approach involving medical intervention and lifestyle modifications, notably dietary adjustments. By adopting dietary changes, individuals can augment their management of these conditions and optimize their overall health and well-being.

Categories of cardiopulmonary disease

Chronic obstructive pulmonary disease (COPD) Obstructed airflow and breathing difficulties are symptoms of COPD, a chronic inflammatory lung disease. COPD may be classified into two main categories: chronic bronchitis and emphysema. The leading cause of chronic obstructive pulmonary disease is smoking. The inability to breathe easily is a symptom of COPD, a chronic inflammatory lung disease. This disease worsens with time since it is progressive. Chronic obstructive pulmonary disease (COPD) is a group of lung illnesses that includes chronic bronchitis and emphysema.

Inflammation of the airways causes a persistent cough accompanied by mucus production; this condition is known as chronic bronchitis. Shortness of breath and other breathing difficulties are symptoms of emphysema, a condition in which the air sacs in the lungs get destroyed. Both of these issues narrow air passages and lessen the amount of oxygen that reaches the lungs, making it more difficult to breathe.

Although cigarette smoking is the primary cause of COPD, other factors such as exposure to air pollution, secondhand smoke, and workplace dust and chemicals can play a role in the disease's progression. COPD symptoms include shortness of breath, wheezing, chest tightness, persistent coughing, and extreme fatigue.

Although there is currently no cure for COPD, treatment can help alleviate symptoms and boost quality of life. Options for treatment range from not smoking to pulmonary rehabilitation to medication to oxygen therapy to, in extreme cases, surgery. Changes in lifestyle, including exercise and a healthy diet, can also aid in the management of COPD symptoms and general health. Managing COPD and preventing further lung damage requires an early diagnosis and treatment.

Asthma

As the airways become inflamed and narrowed, asthma sufferers experience difficulty breathing, wheezing, and coughing on a regular basis. Pollen, dust, and pollution in the air, as well as physical exertion and emotional stress, are all potential precipitating factors. A chronic respiratory condition that affects the airways and makes it difficult to breathe is asthma. It's a widespread problem that can manifest itself in mild to severe forms in persons of all ages.

Asthma's primary symptoms include:

1. Wheezing: a high-pitched whistling sound during respiration

2. Breathing problems (i.e., shortness of breath, difficulty breathing, and fatigue)

3. Tightness or pressure in the chest (sometimes known as "chest tightness").

4. Coughing: Particularly in the wee hours of the night or the morning

Inflammation and narrowing of the airways cause asthma, and this can be triggered by a number of different things.

1. Pollen, dust mites, animal dander, and mold are all examples of allergens.

2. Irritants: things like smoke, pollution, or overpowering scents

3. Respiratory infections, such the common cold or the flu,

4. Physical activity, in particular when the weather is cold or dry

5. Psychic tension

Asthma treatment often consists of a combination of medications and behavioral modifications. Among the most often prescribed drugs for asthma treatment are:

1. Inhaled corticosteroids: for minimizing airway inflammation

2. To ease breathing, bronchodilators work by loosening the muscles that surround the airways.

3. Inhalers of a Variety of Substances at Once: Cholesterol and Bronchodilator Smokers

4. Reducing inflammation and warding off symptoms using leukotriene modifiers.

5. Immune modulators are used to lessen the body's reaction to allergens and stop inflammation from occurring.

Asthma symptoms can be managed with a combination of medication and lifestyle adjustments, such as:

1. Asthma attacks can be avoided with careful identification and avoidance of potential triggers.

2. Frequent exercise can improve lung function and lessen asthma symptoms.

3. Keeping a healthy weight: being overweight might exacerbate asthma symptoms.

4. Adequate sleep is important since lack of it might bring on asthma attacks.

5. Managing stress: For some people, stress is a trigger for asthma attacks.

6. Monitoring symptoms: Asthma attacks can be avoided by keeping track of symptoms and modifying medication as needed.

Talk to your doctor about getting a proper diagnosis and treatment plan if you suspect you have asthma.

Hypertension in the lungs

Pulmonary hypertension is a kind of hypertension that causes strain on the pulmonary and right coronary arteries. Heart failure can occur as a result of underlying illnesses such as pulmonary disease, sleep apnea, or genetic factors. The arteries of the lungs and the right side of the heart are negatively impacted by pulmonary hypertension (PH), a kind of high blood pressure. Pulmonary hypertension causes the arteries in the lungs to narrow or get blocked, reducing blood flow to the lungs. This causes the right side of the heart to work harder to pump blood into the lungs, which in turn increases pressure in the pulmonary arteries. This increased workload can weaken the heart over time, eventually leading to heart failure.

Many underlying conditions, such as those listed below, can lead to PH.

1. Chronic obstructive pulmonary disease (COPD), pulmonary fibrosis, and sleep apnea are all lung illnesses.

2. Congenital heart defects, heart valve disease, and heart failure are all heart diseases.

3. Pulmonary embolisms.

4. Diseases affecting the connective tissues, such as scleroderma or Lupus.

5. Constant illness of the liver.

6. Drugs and specific medications.

Shortness of breath, weariness, chest pain, dizziness, and fainting can all be signs of PH. Many people with PH, however, don't know they have it until the condition has progressed and they start to experience symptoms. ECHOcardiography, pulmonary function tests, and cardiac catheterization are only few of the tests used to diagnose PH.

The treatment for PH is dependent on the underlying cause and severity of the disease. Certain drugs can assist relax the blood vessels in the lungs and improve blood flow, while others can aid in reducing fluid buildup in the body. In extreme circumstances, surgical intervention or a lung transplant may be required. Patients with PH should maintain close communication with their healthcare providers in order to effectively manage their condition and avoid complications.

Coronary artery disease (CAD)

Coronary artery disease (CAD) is a condition in which the coronary arteries, which supply blood to the heart, narrow or become blocked. Chest discomfort, shortness of breath, and even a heart attack might result from this. Coronary artery disease (CAD) occurs when plaque builds up in the arteries supplying blood to the heart, narrowing or blocking them. Plaque is a waxy material composed of cholesterol, fat, and other substances that can accumulate on the inside walls of the arteries over time, causing blockages and other health problems.

When blood flow to the heart is restricted due to narrowed or clogged arteries, symptoms such as chest pain, shortness of breath, and exhaustion can develop. A heart attack might occur if the blockage is particularly severe or if a blood clot forms.

There are a number of risk factors that might lead to coronary artery disease.

Increased blood pressure

- Hypercholesterolemia
- Smoking
- Diabetes

Family history of cardiovascular disease

- Becoming older (risk increases with age)

Medications to decrease blood pressure, cholesterol, or prevent blood clots may be used in conjunction with lifestyle changes such as regular exercise, a nutritious diet, and quitting smoking. Medical procedures such as angioplasy or bypass surgery may be required to unblock arteries in some patients.

Adopting good behaviors like frequent exercise, a nutritious diet, maintaining a healthy weight, and managing chronic conditions like high blood pressure and diabetes can help lower the chance of developing coronary artery disease.

Chronic cardiac insufficiency (CHF)

When the heart cannot pump enough blood to fulfill the body's needs, congestive heart failure (CHF) occurs. Shortness of breath, fatigue, and swelling can result from fluid buildup in the lungs and other organs. Chronic heart failure (CHF) occurs when the heart is unable to pump an adequate amount of blood to provide the body's metabolic demands. Shortness of breath, fatigue, and swelling in the legs and ankles are all symptoms that can result from a buildup of fluid in the lungs and other tissues.

There are a number of risk factors for developing CHF, and these include:

As the arteries supplying blood to the heart muscle become constricted or blocked, the heart's pumping power weakens. This condition is known as coronary artery disease.

Causes the heart to work harder to pump blood, which can lead to congestive heart failure. • High blood pressure.

The heart's muscle becomes weak or enlarged in cardiomyopathy, limiting the heart's ability to pump blood effectively.

Diseases of the heart's valves can make the heart work harder to pump blood, which can lead to congestive heart failure.

Medication, lifestyle adjustments, and even surgery may all play a role in treating congestive heart failure (CHF). You can take diuretics to prevent fluid buildup, angiotensin-converting enzyme inhibitors to reduce blood pressure, and beta-blockers to enhance heart function.

Changing your lifestyle to include a heart-healthy diet, regular exercise, giving up smoking, and cutting back on alcohol are all possibilities. Surgery may be required to repair or replace damaged heart valves or to bypass blocked arteries.

Although CHF is a severe condition, many people are able to live full and active lives with the help of treatment and management. You and your healthcare provider should collaborate closely to create a personalized treatment plan tailored to your needs and goals.

Arrhythmia

The heart can beat too quickly, too slowly, or irregularly due to arrhythmia, an abnormal cardiac rhythm. Several things might contribute to this, such as underlying heart disease, high blood pressure, and unhealthy habits. Arrhythmia is a condition characterized by abnormal or irregular heartbeat. The heart normally beats in a steady rhythm, triggered by a predetermined sequence of electrical signals that causes the muscle to constrict and pump blood throughout the body. People with arrhythmia have an irregular heartbeat, which can cause a variety of symptoms and health problems.

Symptoms of asthma include, but are not limited to the following:

1. A resting heart rate of above 100 beats per minute is considered to be tachycardia.

2. Bradycardia is characterized by a resting heart rate of less than 60 beats per minute.

3. The rapid, irregular heartbeat of atrial fibrillation can lead to dizziness, fatigue, and shortness of breath.

4. A life-threatening arrhythmia that can lead to cardiac arrest and death is ventricular fibrillation.

Heart disease, high blood pressure, diabetes, stress, and certain medications can all contribute to arrhythmia. Some forms of arrhythmia are asymptomatic, while others can cause serious symptoms such chest discomfort, dizziness, fainting, and difficulty breathing.

The kind and severity of an arrhythmia determine the treatment options available. Certain cases of arrhythmia may not necessitate treatment, while others may necessitate medication, lifestyle changes, or medical procedures like catheter ablation or implantable devices like pacemakers or defibrillators.

In some people, avoiding or controlling arrhythmia is as simple as adopting healthier habits like giving up cigarettes, cutting back on alcohol, eating right, and getting regular exercise. A specific treatment plan for arrhythmia based on individual needs and health concerns should be developed in collaboration with a healthcare specialist.

Lung fibroids

Damage to the lungs from pulmonary fibrosis causes breathing problems and a decreased oxygen supply to the body. Exposure to environmental toxins, radiation therapy, and certain medications can all contribute to this condition. Pulmonary fibrosis is a medical condition that results in scarring or fibrous tissue in the lungs. This scarring can hinder lung function, leading to issues with breathing and a lower oxygen supply to the body. Exposure to environmental irritants, infections, autoimmune disorders, and even certain medications have all been linked to the development of pulmonary fibromatosis.

Pulmonary fibrillation symptoms include shortness of breath, a persistent dry cough, fatigue, chest pain, and unexplained weight loss. Typically, a medical history, physical exam, chest x-rays, and other imaging tests all work together to arrive at a diagnosis of pulmonary fibromatosis.

Possible treatments for pulmonary fibrosis range from drugs to lessen inflammation and scarring to oxygen therapy, pulmonary rehabilitation, and even lung transplantation in extreme situations. It is crucial to collaborate closely with a healthcare provider in order to create a treatment plan that is tailored to the individual's unique requirements and health background. These are only a few examples of cardiovascular diseases. Important strategies to improve heart and lung health include stopping smoking, keeping up with a healthy diet and exercise routine, and managing stress. These should all be discussed in detail with your healthcare professional.

The impact of cardiovascular disease on the absorption and utilization of nutrients.

The realm of cardiopulmonary diseases encompasses a spectrum of conditions, including heart failure, pulmonary hypertension, chronic obstructive pulmonary disease (COPD), and asthma. Each of these conditions can significantly impact the body's ability to absorb and utilize nutrients, presenting multifaceted challenges to nutritional health.

1. Oxygen Deficiency and Nutrient Absorption: In conditions such as coronary heart disease, oxygen deficiency is a prevalent concern. This deficiency can impair the body's capacity to absorb and utilize nutrients efficiently. Without adequate

oxygen, cellular function is compromised, hindering nutrient utilization.

2. Loss of Appetite: Cardiopulmonary diseases often coincide with a loss of appetite, making it challenging to consume sufficient nutrients. This loss of appetite can lead to malnutrition and a weakened immune system, exacerbating the effects of the underlying illness.

3. Increased Metabolic Demands: Cardiac diseases can elevate the body's metabolic demands, indicating a heightened need for fuel and nutrients to maintain normal function. When the body's resources cannot meet these increased demands, malnutrition becomes more likely.

4. Medication Interference: Several medications used to manage cardiac illnesses may interfere with the body's ability to absorb and utilize nutrients. Diuretics, for example, can lead to the excretion of vital electrolytes such as potassium and magnesium, essential for muscle function and heart health.

5. Gastrointestinal Symptoms: Cardiac illnesses can manifest gastrointestinal symptoms like nausea, vomiting, and diarrhea, further compromising nutrient absorption and utilization. Medications prescribed to address the underlying condition may also induce these symptoms as side effects.

Cardiovascular diseases can disrupt nutrient absorption and utilization through various mechanisms, including reduced oxygen delivery, decreased appetite, heightened metabolic demands, medication interactions, and gastrointestinal issues. Individuals living with cardiac diseases should collaborate closely with their healthcare providers and registered dietitians to ensure they meet their dietary requirements to support overall health and well-being. Through personalized dietary interventions and medical management, individuals can optimize their nutritional status and mitigate the impact of cardiopulmonary illnesses on their health.

CHAPTER 2
DIETARY NEEDS FOR PATIENTS WITH CARDIOPULMONARY DISEASE

Heart and lung conditions, such as coronary artery disease, congestive heart failure, and chronic obstructive pulmonary disease, are frequently grouped under the umbrella term cardiopulmonary disease (COPD). The nutritional requirements for individuals with cardiopulmonary disease may vary depending on the specific nature of their condition, as well as factors like age, gender, and overall health status. While the dietary needs of individuals with cardiopulmonary disease can be diverse, there exist several overarching dietary guidelines that can offer valuable support and enhance overall health:

1. Moderate Salt Intake: Reducing salt intake is advisable as excessive salt consumption may exacerbate symptoms of cardiopulmonary disease by contributing to fluid retention and elevated blood pressure. Patients with cardiopulmonary disease typically benefit from maintaining a daily salt intake ranging from 1,500 to 2,300 milligrams.

2. Increase Potassium Consumption: Counteracting the effects of sodium on blood pressure can be achieved by incorporating more potassium-rich foods into the diet. Potassium is essential for proper heart and muscle function and can be found abundantly in fruits, vegetables, legumes, and low-fat dairy products.

3. Adopt a Heart-Healthy Diet: Embracing a heart-healthy eating pattern can confer numerous

benefits for individuals with cardiovascular disease, including inflammation reduction, blood pressure improvement, and cholesterol reduction. Such a dietary approach emphasizes the consumption of nutrient-dense foods such as fruits, vegetables, whole grains, lean proteins, and unsaturated fats.

4. Maintain a Healthy Weight: Managing body weight is crucial as being overweight or obese can exacerbate symptoms of cardiopulmonary illness and elevate the risk of complications. Sustaining a healthy weight has been shown to promote overall health and reduce the risk of cardiovascular events.

5. Ensure Adequate Hydration: Patients with cardiovascular disease should prioritize hydration

to prevent dehydration, which can exacerbate breathing difficulties. Adequate fluid intake helps thin mucus, facilitating easier clearance of the airways.

6. Avoid Alcohol and Tobacco: Steering clear of alcohol and cigarette smoke is paramount as they can exacerbate symptoms of heart disease and increase the risk of complications. Quitting smoking and reducing alcohol consumption can have positive effects on overall health and lower the risk of cardiovascular events.

7. Consider Supplementation: Some individuals with cardiovascular disease may benefit from taking supplements such as omega-3 fatty acids, vitamin D, and magnesium. However, it is essential to consult with a healthcare provider

before initiating any supplementation regimen to ensure compatibility with existing medications and mitigate potential risks.

By adhering to these comprehensive dietary guidelines, individuals with cardiopulmonary disease can optimize their nutritional intake, promote heart and lung health, and enhance overall well-being.

The significance of dietary interventions in managing cardiopulmonary diseases.

Diseases affecting the heart and lungs present significant health challenges, yet their management can be significantly enhanced through careful attention to dietary choices.

Conditions such as heart disease, stroke, chronic obstructive pulmonary disease (COPD), asthma, and pulmonary hypertension fall within this category, each demanding tailored nutritional approaches for optimal management.

A well-balanced diet plays a pivotal role in managing cardiovascular diseases by:

1. Mitigating the risk of cardiovascular diseases by prioritizing a diet rich in fruits, vegetables, whole grains, lean proteins, and healthy fats. Given that cardiovascular disease stands as the leading cause of mortality globally, dietary interventions hold immense promise in prevention and management.

2. Controlling blood pressure levels, as hypertension significantly heightens the risk of

cardiovascular diseases, stroke, and related complications. A diet low in sodium and high in potassium has demonstrated efficacy in blood pressure management.

3. Managing blood sugar levels through a healthy diet comprising complex carbohydrates and fiber, given that diabetes serves as a risk factor for cardiovascular disease.

4. Supporting weight maintenance, as obesity escalates the likelihood of developing cardiac diseases. Thus, a nutritious diet aids in weight regulation, fostering overall cardiovascular health.

5. Addressing inflammation, a crucial factor in the onset of cardiopulmonary illnesses. Dietary strategies involving anti-inflammatory foods such

as fruits, vegetables, nuts, and fatty fish help mitigate inflammation, thereby promoting cardiovascular wellness.

6. Enhancing lung function and reducing the risk of lung diseases through a diet abundant in antioxidants like vitamins C and E, as well as omega-3 fatty acids.

Nutrition emerges as a cornerstone in the management of cardiovascular diseases. Adopting a balanced diet replete with a diverse array of fruits, vegetables, whole grains, lean proteins, and healthy fats holds promise in not only reducing the risk of developing certain diseases but also alleviating their associated symptoms, thereby fostering improved health outcomes and overall well-being.

Describing the distinctive nutritional needs of individuals afflicted with cardiopulmonary ailments.

Heart and lung diseases collectively fall under the category known as cardiopulmonary diseases. Among the various conditions encompassed within this classification are coronary heart disease (CHD), congestive heart failure (CHF), chronic obstructive pulmonary disease (COPD), and asthma. These disorders can significantly impact an individual's nutritional requirements, affecting their body's ability to absorb nutrients, increasing the risk of malnutrition, and potentially leading to the development of other health complications.

Individuals with cardiopulmonary diseases have distinct and specialized nutritional needs that should be addressed:

1. Protein intake: Maintaining adequate protein intake is crucial for preserving muscle mass and promoting healing, particularly for individuals with cardiovascular disease. Lean meats, poultry, fish, beans, and tofu are all excellent sources of protein.

2. Fluid balance: Certain medications used to treat cardiac diseases may cause fluid retention or dehydration. Therefore, it is essential to maintain a healthy fluid balance to prevent complications such as swelling and electrolyte imbalances. Monitoring fluid intake and output is crucial for managing these conditions effectively.

3. Sodium restriction: Individuals with cardiovascular diseases are generally advised to limit their salt intake to prevent fluid retention and hypertension. Reducing the consumption of processed foods, canned soups, and salty snacks can help achieve this goal.

4. Potassium intake: Potassium is an essential mineral that helps counteract the negative effects of sodium on blood pressure. Foods rich in potassium, such as bananas, sweet potatoes, spinach, and yogurt, should be included in the diet.

5. Omega-3 fatty acids: Omega-3 fatty acids offer numerous benefits for heart health and may help reduce inflammation throughout the body.

Sources of omega-3s include fatty fish like salmon, walnuts, chia seeds, and flaxseed oil.

6. Antioxidants: Antioxidants play a crucial role in reducing inflammation and protecting the body from damage caused by free radicals. Foods rich in antioxidants include fruits, vegetables, nuts, and whole grains.

7. Vitamin D: Adequate vitamin D levels are essential for bone health and may also play a role in preventing heart disease. Individuals with cardiac disorders may be at a higher risk of vitamin D insufficiency due to limited sun exposure and poor nutrition. Foods such as fatty fish, egg yolks, and fortified products like milk and cereal are good sources of vitamin D.

Collaborating with a healthcare provider or registered dietitian to develop an individualized nutrition plan tailored to the unique needs of individuals with cardiovascular disease is paramount. This personalized approach ensures that dietary recommendations align with specific health goals and medical considerations, optimizing overall health and well-being.

CHAPTER 3
FOODS TO AVOID IF YOU HAVE CARDIOPULMONARY DISEASE

The term "cardiopulmonary disease" encompasses a spectrum of medical conditions that affect both the heart and lungs, constituting a complex interplay of physiological disturbances. Among these conditions are coronary artery disease, heart failure, chronic obstructive pulmonary disease (COPD), and various others. It is imperative to recognize the pivotal role of dietary habits in managing these conditions effectively and mitigating the likelihood of complications. Certain dietary choices have the potential to exacerbate symptoms and elevate the risk of cardiovascular events and respiratory disorders, necessitating careful consideration and modification of dietary patterns for individuals grappling with cardiopulmonary ailments.

1. Fried and processed foods, notorious for their high content of unhealthy fats, salt, and sugar, pose a significant risk to cardiovascular health. Moreover, certain foods high in trans fats, prevalent in processed and fried items, have been implicated in the pathogenesis of heart disease, emphasizing the importance of minimizing their consumption.

2. Diets rich in sodium are associated with fluid retention, imposing additional strain on the heart and lungs. Excessive salt intake can elevate blood pressure levels, thereby exacerbating the risk of cardiovascular disease. Individuals with cardiopulmonary conditions are advised to adhere

to a sodium intake of no more than 2,300 milligrams per day to optimize their health outcomes.

3. Consumption of red meat in large quantities may elevate the risk of heart disease due to its saturated fat content. Additionally, it can exacerbate COPD symptoms by contributing to pulmonary inflammation and oxidative stress.

4. Dairy products, particularly full-fat varieties like cheese and cream, contain high levels of saturated fats that can elevate cholesterol levels and heighten the risk of heart disease. Individuals with COPD may experience digestive issues and worsened respiratory symptoms if they also have lactose intolerance.

5. Sugar-sweetened beverages, including soda, sports drinks, sweetened tea, and flavored coffee, are laden with calories and sugar, contributing to weight gain and an increased risk of heart disease and diabetes. Moreover, certain beverages can exacerbate COPD symptoms by promoting airway inflammation and mucus production.

6. Alcohol consumption can elevate blood pressure and lipid levels, both of which increase the risk of cardiovascular disease. Furthermore, alcohol can exacerbate COPD symptoms by inflaming the lungs and reducing lung capacity.

Individuals with cardiovascular disease should eschew these dietary culprits and instead focus on consuming a wholesome, balanced diet replete with fruits, vegetables, whole grains, lean proteins, and healthy fats. Adequate hydration is paramount, and individuals should limit their caffeine intake as it may interfere with medication efficacy and potentially induce dehydration. Consulting with a healthcare provider or registered dietitian is advised to formulate a tailored nutrition plan aligned with specific health goals and preferences.

The way specific foods can worsen symptoms or increase the likelihood of complications.

Providing an exhaustive description of how certain foods might exacerbate symptoms or heighten the risk of health issues necessitates a nuanced understanding of the specific dietary items under consideration. While it's challenging to delve into specifics without context, we can explore several instances more broadly:

1. High-Sodium Diets: These are generally discouraged for individuals with hypertension, heart disease, or other cardiovascular conditions due to their potential to induce dangerous spikes in blood pressure.

2. High-Sugar Foods: Consumption of foods high in sugar can lead to elevated blood sugar levels, posing challenges for individuals with diabetes. Prolonged high blood sugar levels may increase the risk of diabetes-related complications such as nerve damage and kidney disease over time.

3. Saturated and Trans Fats: Consuming foods rich in saturated and trans fats has been associated

with elevated levels of LDL (low-density lipoprotein) cholesterol, often referred to as "bad" cholesterol. Elevated LDL levels are known to increase the risk of cardiovascular disease.

4. Food Allergens and Intolerances: Certain foods can exacerbate symptoms in individuals with food allergies or intolerances, manifesting as gastrointestinal distress, skin rashes, or breathing difficulties. Common allergens include tree nuts, seafood, milk products, and wheat.

5. Fast Food and Processed Foods: Regular consumption of these types of meals has been linked to an increased risk of developing various serious health conditions, including obesity, Type 2 diabetes, and heart disease. These foods typically contain high levels of calories, sodium, sugar, and

unhealthy fats while being low in fiber, vitamins, and minerals.

A healthy diet should primarily comprise whole, nutrient-dense foods such as fruits, vegetables, whole grains, lean meats, and healthy fats. If you have specific dietary needs or health concerns, seeking guidance from a doctor or certified dietitian to formulate a personalized nutrition plan is advisable. Their expertise can help tailor a diet that addresses your individual requirements and promotes overall well-being.

CHAPTER 4
FOODS TO INCLUDE IN A DIET FOR CARDIOVASCULAR DISEASE

Diseases affecting the heart and lungs stand as formidable adversaries in the realm of global health, accounting for a significant portion of mortality and disability worldwide. Fortunately, the risk of complications stemming from these conditions can be mitigated, and their management optimized, through the adoption of a health-conscious diet. Herein lies a comprehensive array of dietary recommendations aimed at combatting cardiovascular disease and supporting lung health:

1. Embrace a Spectrum of Fruits and Vegetables: Harness the nutritional prowess of a diverse array of fruits and vegetables, which abound with essential vitamins, minerals, fiber, and

antioxidants. Cultivate a vibrant palette of colors and textures by incorporating an assortment of produce into your meals, including leafy greens, succulent berries, tangy citrus fruits, and robust vegetables like broccoli and Brussels sprouts.

2. Opt for Whole Grains: Champion the cause of whole grains, revered for their complex carbohydrates and fiber content, both of which play pivotal roles in regulating blood sugar levels and mitigating inflammation. Prioritize foods crafted from whole grains such as bread, pasta, rice, oats, and quinoa to furnish your body with enduring nourishment.

3. Lean Protein Selections: Elevate your protein intake with lean sources such as fish, skinless poultry, and lentils, which deliver vital amino

acids sans the burden of excessive saturated fat or cholesterol.

4. Harness the Power of Omega-3 Fatty Acids: Unveil the therapeutic potential of omega-3 fatty acids, abundant in fatty fish like salmon, which have been heralded for their anti-inflammatory properties and heart-health benefits. Extend your repertoire of healthful fats by incorporating nuts, seeds, avocados, and olive oil into your dietary regimen.

5. Mindful Dairy Consumption: Exercise prudence in selecting low-fat or fat-free dairy products to circumvent the pitfalls of excessive saturated fat intake. Dairy products serve as rich sources of calcium and other essential nutrients, contributing to your overall nutritional profile.

6. Embrace Flavorful Herbs and Spices: Infuse your culinary creations with an explosion of flavor using herbs and spices, thus obviating the need for excess salt, which can exert a deleterious impact on blood pressure. Explore the multifaceted culinary potential of Grocery List such as garlic, ginger, turmeric, and cinnamon.

7. Prioritize Hydration: Maintain optimal hydration levels, a cornerstone of good health, particularly for individuals grappling with cardiovascular disease. Aim to consume a minimum of eight glasses of water daily while curtailing your intake of sugary beverages and caffeinated drinks.

In tandem with integrating these dietary essentials into your daily fare, it is equally imperative to exercise vigilance in limiting or eschewing foods that might heighten your susceptibility to complications. Steer clear of processed meals, sugary beverages, and excesses of salt and saturated fat. Collaborate with your healthcare provider or a registered dietitian to craft a tailored cardiopulmonary disease diet plan attuned to your unique requirements and aspirations. Through mindful dietary choices and strategic guidance, you can embark on a journey towards enhanced cardiovascular and pulmonary wellness.

Ways in which these food items can mitigate symptoms and reduce risk factors.

Providing a comprehensive response necessitates delving into the specific culinary options you have in mind. However, in a broad sense, the adoption of a nourishing and well-balanced diet holds the promise of symptom amelioration and the reduction of complications across various health conditions.

A dietary regimen rich in fruits and vegetables, whole grains, lean proteins, and healthy fats has emerged as a cornerstone in the quest for enhanced health outcomes. This dietary paradigm has been closely associated with diminished rates of cardiovascular diseases, diabetes, and several types of cancers. Fruits and vegetables, in particular, brim with anti-inflammatory nutrients such as vitamins, minerals, antioxidants, and fiber, which collectively wield the power to quell inflammation and fortify the immune system.

Moreover, certain foods and nutrients have demonstrated therapeutic efficacy in addressing specific maladies. For instance, fatty fish like salmon, mackerel, and sardines serve as rich reservoirs of omega-3 fatty acids, renowned for their anti-inflammatory properties and cardiovascular benefits. Probiotic-rich foods such as yogurt and kefir contribute to digestive health and bolster immune function. High-fiber foods like beans, lentils, and whole grains play pivotal roles in regulating blood sugar levels and promoting digestive well-being.

By incorporating a diverse array of nutrient-dense foods into your dietary repertoire, you can potentially alleviate symptoms and mitigate the risk of complications across a spectrum of health issues. However, for personalized guidance tailored to your unique needs and health concerns, seeking counsel from a medical professional or registered dietitian is highly advisable. Their expertise can illuminate the path toward optimal health and wellness, ensuring that your dietary choices align harmoniously with your health objectives and aspirations.

CHAPTER 5
CARDIOPULMONARY DIET RECIPES

BREAKFAST

Hearty Raspberry Pancakes

Grocery List

1/2 cup whole wheat flour

1/2 cup whole wheat pastry flour

1/4 cup ground flax seed

1/4 cup granulated sugar

1 teaspoon baking powder

1 pinch salt

1 1/2 teaspoons vanilla extract

1 tablespoon canola oil

1 cup low-fat milk

1/2 cup walnuts

3/4 cup black raspberries (may substitute small red raspberries)

Instructions

Chop the walnuts into a coarse meal.

In a medium mixing bowl, whisk together the flours, flax seed, sugar, baking powder and salt.

Add the vanilla, canola oil and milk, stirring until completely mixed together.

Fold in the raspberries and walnuts.

Preheat a greased skillet or griddle over medium heat. When a drop of water sizzles when it is flicked onto the skillet, you are ready to make some pancakes.

Pour about 1/2 cup of batter onto the skillet and allow to cook for 2-3 minutes. When the edges are set, flip the pancake and cook for another minute or two until both sides of the pancake are browned. Remove to a plate to partially cool, and repeat with the rest of the batter.

Hearty Almond Pancakes

Grocery List

1/2 cup almond flour

1/2 cup oat flour

1/4 cup ground flax

1/4 cup coconut, unsweetened

1/2 teaspoon baking soda and baking powder

1/2 teaspoon salt

1 cup milk + 1 teaspoon lemon

2 tablespoons canola oil

1 teaspoon vanilla

1 egg

Instructions

Combine dry ingredients together. set aside

In a different bowl, add lemon juice to milk. Add in remaining wet Grocery List and combined into dry. Do not overmix

Let the batter sit for 15 minutes - it will really thicken up.

Cook pancakes over medium heat on a greased pan. Can serve with homemade nut butter.

Hearty Oatmeal Bread

Grocery List

1 quart plus 1/2 cup boiling water

2 cups rolled oats - NOT the quick kind

1/2 cup raw wheat germ

2 teaspoons sea salt

10 ounces unsulphured molasses (Grandma's yellow label)

1/3 cup safflower oil

2 tablespoons dry yeast (I use SAF)

12 cups (approximately) stone ground whole wheat flour

Instructions

Pour boiling water over oats, wheat germ, molasses, oil and salt in a very large bowl. Cool to lukewarm. Stir in yeast to dissolve. Then add flour to form a stiff dough. Knead well. (This bread will take a LOT of kneading, so be patient. The longer you can knead it, the more fabulous the texture will be.)

Place in greased bowl and seal the top with oiled plastic wrap to rise until double (at least 1 hour).

Heat the oven to 350 degrees F. When the dough has doubled in bulk, punch down (get most of the air out). Form into four equal loaves. Put into 9x5-inch loaf pans. Cover pans with plastic wrap. Let rise until nearly double. (Unless your kitchen is exceptionally warm, this will take about 40 minutes to an hour – but watch them.)

Bake for 1 hour until the loaves "tap hollow." (For a softer crust, put a pan of water on the lower shelf and cover each loaf with a "tent" of aluminum foil (shiny side in). Remove from pans and cool on cake racks.

Hearty Baked Oatmeal

Grocery List

2 large eggs

3/4 cup brown sugar

1/3 cup unsalted butter, melted and cooled slightly

1.5 teaspoons baking powder

1.5 teaspoons vanilla extract

3 teaspoons ground flax seed

1 teaspoon cinnamon

1 teaspoon nutmeg

1 pinch salt

1 cup

2 tablespoons milk

1/2 cup shredded sweetened coconut, toasted

3 cups rolled oats

Toasted walnuts, cranberries, or any assortment of toppings you like

Instructions

Lightly grease an 8?x8? baking dish.

Mix eggs and brown sugar in the bottom of the dish, whisking to remove lumps. Add melted butter and carefully whisk to combine.

Add baking powder, vanilla, ground flax seed, cinnamon, nutmeg and salt directly to the dish and whisk well. Carefully add the milk and stir to combine.

Add the toasted coconut and oats and carefully fold into the mixture, making sure everything is combined really well. Cover the dish with plastic wrap and refrigerate over night.

The next morning, preheat the oven to 350 degrees and bake the oatmeal for approximately 45 minutes, or until the edges are brown.

Remove from oven and let cool for a few minutes. Then cut yourself a piece, top it with toasted walnuts and dried cherries, and pour some warm milk over the top. Enjoy!

Hearty Quiche

Grocery List

1- 9" unbaked pie shell

6 strps bacon, cooked crisp, crumble and set aside

1 large onion, chopped fine

1-1/2 cups grated natural Swiss cheese (6 oz.) or Gruyre

1/2 cup chopped ham

1 medium potato, cut to 1/4 to 1/2 inch cubed

1/2 cup sliced mushrooms

1-10 ounces box frozen chopped spinach, very well drained

2 tablespoons flour

4 eggs

2 cups Half & Half

1 teaspoon salt

1/4 teaspoon pepper

1/2 teaspoon Oregano

1/2 teaspoon Rosemary

2 tablespoons Sour Cream

4 tablespoons grated Parmessan Cheece

Instructions

In pan bacon was cooked in, drain off all but one tablespoon of bacon drippings. Cook onion and potatoes until soft. Add ham and mushrooms and heat through, remove from heat.

Mix together in a large bowl, 2 tablespoons flour, 4 eggs, 2 cups Half & Half, 1 teaspoon salt, 1/4 teaspoon pepper, 1/2 teaspoon oregano, 1/2 teaspoon Rosemary, mix well. Add the grated cheese, bacon, ham, onion, potatoes, mushrooms, grated Parmessan cheese, sour cream and well drained chopped spinach. (Drain spinach by squeezing it very well with your hands.) Mix all Grocery List well and pour into unbaked pie shell.

Bake at 350° for 40 to 45 minutes, or until puffed and brown. Cool 30 minutes before cutting into 8 wedges.

Heart-Healthy Vanilla Blueberry Muffins

Grocery List

1/4 cup unsweetened applesauce

1 ripe banana, mashed

1 cup wheat bran

1/4 cup almond meal

1/4 cup hemp hearts

1 cup blueberries (fresh or frozen)

1/2 cup water

2 tablespoons melted virgin coconut oil

2 tablespoons vanilla extract

1 teaspoon cinnamon

3/4 teaspoon baking soda

1/3 cup water

Instructions

Preheat oven to 350 F.

Mix all the Grocery List in a big bowl.

Pour mixture into cupcake tins.

Bake for 12–15 minutes, and check with a fork or toothpick to see if they're done.

Heart Healthy Breakfast: Avocado Toast

Grocery List

2 slices of your favorite seedy whole grain bread, lightly toasted

1 small avocado, cut in half, pit removed

1 beefsteak tomato, sliced

2 Persian cucumbers, skin on, ends trimmed, long thin ribbons made by a vegetable peeler

1/4 small red onion, thinly sliced

1 teaspoon freshly squeezed lemon juice

Extra Virgin olive oil, for drizzling

salt and pepper to taste

red pepper flakes to taste

Instructions

Place the toasted bread on a cutting board. Using a butter knife, scoop out some avocado flesh and spread evenly on each toast, covering the whole area. Drizzle 1/2 teaspoon lemon juice on each toast.

Place 1-2 two tomato slices on top of avocado.

Place sliced onion on top of the tomato.

Gently weave the cucumber ribbons on top making a lattice pattern.

Drizzle lightly with olive oil. Sprinkle with red pepper flakes. Season to taste with salt and pepper.

Seitan Burritos

Grocery List:

1 can refried black beans,

1 cup fresh tomato salsa,

1 green bell pepper,

1 package ground seitan,

1 tbsp. extra virgin olive oil,

1 tsp. chili powder,

1 tsp. cumin,

1 tsp. nutritional yeast,

1/2 yellow onion,

4 whole-grain tortilla wraps,

Salt & pepper —healthfood

Instructions

Chop up the onion and green pepper into strips and drop them in a sauté pan with the olive oil over medium heat. Allow the onions and peppers to cook for a few minutes, then add in the ground seitan and stir. Sprinkle in the cumin, chili powder, nutritional yeast, and a dash of salt and black pepper. Mix well and continue to cook for about 5 minutes, stirring frequently. Meanwhile, warm up your tortillas and refried black beans in the oven or microwave. Spread a healthy portion of the beans on each tortilla, top with the sautéed seitan, peppers, and onions, and about a quarter of a cup of salsa. Drizzle a little hot sauce on to taste. Wrap up into a burrito and serve immediately. Tips: Nutritional yeast can be found at your local health food store. Full of protein and B vitamins, it's a healthy spice that adds a rich, cheesy flavor. You can also try adding diced avocado to this dish for a super creamy texture.

Strawberry Rosemary Mojito

Grocery List

The Drink

2 ounces light rum (white rum like Bacardi or Havana Club)

juice of 1/2 a lime

3 tablespoons aromatic rosemary flavored simple syrup

2 ounces club soda

2 strawberries quartered and 1 whole for decoration

5 leaves of rosemary (optional) and 1 sprig for decoration

ice

Aromatic Rosemary Flavored Simple Syrup

1 cup sugar

1 cup water

1 heaping tablespoon of rosemary leaves

Instructions

The Drink

In a large tumbler, squeeze juice of ½ a lime, 3 tablespoons aromatic rosemary flavored simple syrup, 2 strawberries, quartered and muddle, until the strawberries are crushed, leaving a few big bits to release the strawberry flavor.

Pour 2 ounces of rum into the tumbler, fill with ice cubes, top with 2 ounces of soda, and add the rosemary leaves and stir.

Cut the remaining strawberry, lengthwise nearly in half and place on the side of the glass add a sprig of rosemary for the final touch before serving.

Balsamic Fried Eggs

Grocery List

2 tablespoons extra virgin olive oil

2 large eggs

kosher salt and freshly ground black pepper

2 slices toasted hearty bread

1 1/2 tablespoons balsamic vinegar

2 handfuls arugula

Instructions

Add olive oil to an 8 inch skillet over medium heat. When the oil is hot but not at the smoking point, crack open the eggs, one at a time, letting each egg set. Cook for about 25 seconds, keeping the heat at medium. As the eggs puff up, season with salt and pepper. Tilt the pan and baste the top of the yolks with the oil to help them cook. Cook to desired doneness. Place a piece of toast on each plate, top with an egg. Pour off and discard any excess oil and remove any oily residue from the pan. Put the pan back over medium heat. Add the balsamic vinegar and let it sizzle and reduce slightly for a moment or two. Drizzle over the eggs. Garnish with arugula and serve.

Cranberry Ginger Almond Crunch Muffins

Grocery List

0.25 cups rolled old-fashioned oats

0.25 cups slivered almonds

0.25 cups butter, melted

2 tablespoons brown sugar

1 teaspoon ground cinnamon

0.75 cups brown sugar

2 large eggs

0.25 cups heart-healthy oil

0.25 cups milk

1 teaspoon vanilla extract

1.5 cups oat flour (or ground oats)

0.5 cups rolled old-fashioned oats

1.5 teaspoons baking powder

1 teaspoon baking soda

0.5 teaspoons coarse salt

0.5 teaspoons ground ginger

1 cup fresh or frozen cranberries

Instructions

Preheat oven to 350 degrees.

In a small bowl, combine the oats, slivered almonds, butter, brown sugar and cinnamon

In a medium mixing bowl, whisk together brown sugar, eggs, oil, milk and vanilla extract until combined.

In another medium mixing bowl, whisk together oat flour, oats, baking powder, baking soda, salt and ginger. Pour dry Grocery List into the bowl of wet ingredients and whisk together until just combined. Fold in cranberries.

Spoon batter into the wells of a greased 9-cup muffin tin, about ¾ of the way full. Top with a scoop of the oat/almond topping. Bake 18-20 minutes, until toothpick inserted into the center of the muffin comes out clean. Allow to cool.

Basil Goat Cheese Toast with Fresh Peaches

Grocery List

3.5 ounces goat cheese

5 sprigs basil

2 slices hearty bread, thickness is up to your preference

1 ripe peach, sliced thick

honey

Instructions

Remove leaves from basil sprigs, stack them and roll them up, and slice as thinly as you can. Mix this basil with your soft goat cheese. I make up a big batch of this and keep it in the fridge all week.

Toast your bread, spread the basil goat cheese thickly (I usually use about half of the amount this recipe makes). Drizzle honey across the top, and layer on the peaches.

Banana, Blueberry, and Pecan Pancakes

Grocery List

For the batter:

100 grams oats

A good handful of pecan nuts (about 50g), roughly chopped

1 teaspoon baking powder

A pinch of sea salt

1 ripe banana, peeled and mashed

150 milliliters coconut milk or almond milk

A punnet of blueberries (about 200g, or use frozen)

To serve:

2 bananas, peeled and cut into thin slices

A little coconut oil or butter, a few crumbled pecan nuts, lime wedges, and honey or agave syrup

Instructions

First turn the oven to 120°C/fan 100°C/gas 1/2 to keep everything warm.

Blitz the oats until you have a scruffy oat flour. Add to a bowl with the pecans and throw in the baking powder and salt.

Mix the mashed banana with the milk (you can do this by blitzing them together in the food processor, if you like). Beat the banana mixture into the flour and leave the batter to sit for a few minutes.

Heat a non-stick pan on a medium heat, then add the banana slices and fry on both sides in the dry pan until brown and caramelised. Keep warm in the oven.

Put the pan back on a medium heat and add a little coconut oil or butter. Drop in a healthy tablespoonful of batter for each pancake. Once the sides are cooked and bubbles have risen to the top, scatter over a handful of blueberries and flip the pancake over. Cook for another couple of minutes on the other side. The pancakes will stay a little moist in the middle because of the banana, so don't worry. Keep them warm in the oven while you cook the rest.

Serve the pancakes piled with the banana slices. Add some crumbled pecans and a squeeze of lime, and, if you like, a little touch of honey, agave or maple syrup.

Soft-Scrambled Eggs "Alla Gricia"

Grocery List

1/2 tablespoon olive oil

3 ounces guanciale (salt-cured pork jowl), sliced to about 1/8-inch thick and torn into bite sized pieces (you can substitute in bacon if you can't find guanciale)

3 large eggs

1 large pinch of salt

1 tablespoon finely grated pecorino, plus more for serving

1 tablespoon butter, cubed

1 large pinch of freshly ground black pepper, for serving

Instructions

In a small non-stick skillet over medium heat, heat olive oil until glistening and then add the guanciale. Brown the guanciale without jostling it too much, so it crisps up on both sides. This will take about 3 to 5 minutes, and the meat will shrink as its fat renders into the oil. Using a slotted spoon, remove the crispy guanciale and set aside, reserving half the rendered fat and oil in the pan. Let the pan sit off heat to cool while you prepare the eggs.

Crack eggs into a bowl and whisk together with salt and pecorino, just so they're totally homogenous. Add the cubes of butter.

Heat the skillet with the reserved guanciale fat over medium-low until the fat becomes translucent, then pour the egg mixture into the skillet. Using a spatula, stir the eggs every minute or so to encourage large curds to form, turning the heat down to low if they start to cook quickly.

Continue this for about 4 minutes, until curds have formed but the eggs still have a custardy sheen. Move the eggs to a plate (they'll continue to cook a bit), and top with guanciale crisps, a healthy sprinkling of pecorino, and a large pinch of freshly ground black pepper.

Day- After Casserole for a Hearty Breakfast

Grocery List

2 cups leftover meat (turky,beef, pork, chicken, lamb or sausages) chopped in bite-size pieces

2 tablespoons olive oil

1 medium onion diced

1 large or two small leeks (white part) sliced

2 large garlic cloves minced

2-3 medium zucchini unpeeled or 1 large eggplant cut in half and sliced in ¼-inch pieces

2 cups can tomatoes, drained

1 cup good quality red wine

1 cup fresh or frozen peas

¼ teaspoon ground cinnamon

¼ teaspoon nutmeg freshly ground

2 teaspoons salt

½ teaspoon red pepper flakes

1/2 a pound pasta of your choice fresh cooked or leftover (al dente), I like Pappardelle

½ cup grated Parmesan, Romano or Sharp White Cheddar cheese

2-3 tablespoons fresh herbs of your choice(chopped)

Instructions

Brown the meat in oil; add onion, leeks, and salt; sauté until tender. Stir in zucchini, tomatoes, garlic, and wine, cinnamon, nutmeg, and red pepper flakes; sauté for about 10 minutes or until the mixture is reduced in half. Set aside to cool to room temperature.

Meanwhile cook pasta; before draining reserve ½ cup of the cooking liquid. If using leftover pasta, worm it in a double boiler. Gently mix everything together; fold in the fresh peas, chopped herbs, and cheese. If you fill that the mixture needs more moisture, add the reserved cooking liquid.

Taste for seasoning; grease a four-quart casserole baking dish; pour the mixture, smooth-out the top. In a small bowl combine ½ cup Panko breadcrumbs, 1 tablespoon Extra Virgin olive oil and some more grated cheese. Sprinkle over the top and bake for 30 minutes in 400 degrees preheated oven.

LUNCH AND DINNER

Simple Seasoned Adzuki Beans

Grocery List

4 cups dried aduki beans (or pinto or another type of beans)

4 slices preservative-free bacon, sliced into 1 inch pieces- optional; bacon lends a nice smoky saltiness but you can leave out for vegetarian beans

1 teaspoon course sea salt or to taste

1 teaspoon black pepper or to taste

1 teaspoon garlic powder or to taste

1 teaspoon chili powder or to taste

Instructions

If not using aduki beans, it's best to soak your beans overnight in a large pot covered with water. After they have soaked, drain them and rinse several times. If you are using the aduki beans, just go ahead and rinse them.

Place rinsed beans and bacon in a large pot on the stove. Pour water over the beans to cover by 2 inches. Bring to a boil and then reduce the heat to a simmer.

Skim any foam that might rise to the top while cooking, and add additional water (or stock), if there does not seem to be enough liquid.

Cook until the beans are tender, about 1 1/2 hours (or as long as 3 hours for pinto and other beans).

5. Add the sea salt (don't add too much if you've used stock) and pepper, plus the seasonings I

mentioned (or others that you like) to taste. You can serve these in whole wheat or corn tortillas with the toppings of your choice: think grated raw cheese, fresh salsa, guacamole, organic sour cream, etc. Or have some in a bowl with a side of cornbread. Fresh chopped tomato, cucumber, red pepper, and sliced avocado are also wonderful additions.

My favorite healthy way to eat these, though, is this: chop some collard greens very fine, add some olive oil and fresh lime juice, and mix with the beans, veggies, and salsa. Top with some green onions and minced cilantro.

Hearty Spicy Kale and Pork Soup/Stew with White Beans

Grocery List

1 tablespoon olive oil

1 pound boneless pork loin or chops, trimmed and cut into bite-size pieces

Mrs. Dash Table Blend, or salt, to taste

Ground Black Pepper, to taste

1 cup chopped onion

2 garlic cloves, minced

1 teaspoon Hungarian paprika

1 teaspoon Ancho chile powder

1 or 2 pinches of crushed red pepper flakes

1/4 cup red wine

4 Roma (plum) tomatoes, chopped

4 to 5 cups chicken or turkey broth, homemade or low sodium

1 bunch of kale, ribs removed and chopped

1 can of white beans, drained and rinsed

Instructions

Heat the oil in a dutch oven or soup pot on medium high.

Generously season the pork with the Mrs. Dash and black pepper, then add to the pot. Brown the pork on all sides, then remove to a bowl and set aside.

Add the chopped onion to the pot, and cook for about five minutes until starting to soften.

Add the minced garlic, Hungarian paprika, Ancho chile powder and crushed red pepper flakes, and stir for about a minute longer.

Add the red wine and chopped tomatoes, stirring to scrape up any browned bits on the bottom.

Add the broth, then bring to a boil. Add the kale (it looks like a lot, but it all wilts down just like spinach) until it's mixed in, then turn down the heat to a low simmer.

Add the pork back in and the white beans (I used cannellini) and continue simmering until ready to eat.

Hearty Hamburger Helper with Wagyu Beef

Grocery List

2 pounds Double 8 Cattle Company Fullblood Wagyu Ground Beef

2 tablespoons Butter

1 Sweet Onion (chopped)

1 teaspoon Chili Powder

1 teaspoon Paprika

1 teaspoon Garlic Powder

1 pound Orecchiette Pasta

1 Zucchini (grated)

2 cups Beef Broth

1 1/2 cups Whole Milk

1 tablespoon Ketchup

2 cups Shredded Cheddar Cheese

1 bunch Parsley (chopped, to garnish)

Instructions

Tools, Dutch Oven, Wooden Spatula, Grater, Cutting Board

FIRST STEP Take the Fullblood Wagyu ground beef out of the freezer, and place it in the refrigerator 24 hours before starting this recipe.

PREPARING THE HAMBURGER HELPER

Place a Dutch oven over medium-high heat. Add the butter, chopped sweet onion, and Fullblood

Wagyu ground beef to the Dutch oven. Cook the beef until thoroughly browned, while breaking it up with a wooden spatula as you go. Stir in the chili powder, paprika, and garlic powder. Cook for approximately one more minute. Add the Orecchiette pasta and grated zucchini, while mixing. Next, add the beef broth, whole milk, and ketchup. Continue to stir until evenly distributed. Bring the mixture to a boil over high heat. Then reduce the heat, and simmer for about 10 minutes until the pasta is cooked.

FINAL STEPS Stir in the shredded cheddar cheese, and continue to cook until the mixture is very creamy. Divide the hamburger helper between bowls, and garnish with chopped parsley. Serve, and enjoy!

Matelote (Fish Stew)

Grocery List

14 to 16 ounces peeled or unpeeled pearl onions, fresh or frozen and thawed

Extra-virgin olive oil, for sautéing

5 ounces pancetta, cut into lardons (about 1 cup)

8 ounces button mushrooms, halved

1/4 cup cognac

3 cups fish or seafood stock

7 black peppercorns

5 (2-inch) parsley stems

3 thyme sprigs

1 dried bay leaf

1 garlic clove, peeled

1 clove

Kosher salt, to taste

1 (750-milliliter) bottle dry Riesling

20 mussels, scrubbed and debearded

8 ounces skin-on halibut (or monkfish), sliced into hearty chunks

8 ounces skin-on sea bass (or perch), sliced into hearty chunks

8 ounces Arctic char (or salmon), sliced into hearty chunks

12 to 15 U/20 shrimp, peeled and deveined

2 tablespoons all-purpose flour

2 tablespoons unsalted butter, at room temperature

3 tablespoons chopped flat-leaf parsley leaves

1 tablespoon chopped tarragon leaves

Toasted baguette or sourdough, or cooked long noodles

Instructions

If your onions are not peeled, bring a small pot of water to boil. Add the onions and cook for 2 minutes. Drain them in a colander and run under cold water until cool enough to handle. Peel. (If your onions are thawed from frozen and already peeled, skip this skip.)

In a wide pot or Dutch oven over medium-low heat, add a big drizzle of oil and cook the pancetta until crispy, 10 to 12 minutes, stirring occasionally. Use a slotted spoon to transfer the pancetta to a large bowl.

Add the onions to the same pan, agitating the pan to coat them in the hot fat (you can add another drizzle of oil if the pan looks dry). Sauté over medium-low until they start to brown, 5 to 7 minutes, stirring occasionally.

Add the mushrooms and agitate the pan again. Over medium, sauté the mushrooms until golden and soft, about 7 minutes, stirring occasionally.

Add the cognac and reduce almost completely, about 1 minute. Transfer the onions, mushrooms, and any remaining liquid to the bowl of pancetta.

Add the stock to the pot and stir any liquor residue into the stock. Raise the heat to medium.

While that heats up, wrap the peppercorns, parsley stems, thyme sprigs, bay leaf, garlic clove, and clove in a piece of muslin (or extra-fine cheesecloth) and secure with kitchen twine. Add this bouquet garni to the stock, along with ½ teaspoon salt and the wine. Bring to a boil over high heat.

Add the mussels, agitate the pan so they settle into an even later, cover the pot, and lower the heat to medium-high. After about 5 minutes, their shells should have opened. Use a slotted spoon to strain and transfer them to a large bowl. Discard any mussels that haven't opened. Remove and discard the bouquet garni.

Add the pancetta, onions, and mushrooms, plus any accumulated juices to the stock mixture and return to a gentle simmer. Add the halibut and poach for 3 minutes, until the flesh turns fully opaque, lowering the heat as needed so the mixture barely bubbles, then use a slotted spoon to transfer the halibut to the bowl with mussels. Add the sea bass and poach for 2 minutes, until opaque everywhere but in the middle, then transfer to the bowl with mussels. Add the Arctic char and poach for 2 minutes, until opaque everywhere but in the middle, then transfer to the bowl with mussels. Add the shrimp and cook for 2 to 3 minutes, until nearly opaque in the center, then transfer to the bowl with the mussels.

In a small bowl, use a spoon to mash the flour into the butter until fully incorporated—it will resemble a thick paste. Add to the pot and stir regularly for 5 to 7 minutes, until the broth is somewhat thickened.

Taste and adjust the salt as needed. Gently add back all of the fish, mussels, and shrimp and stir to incorporate. Ladle into wide shallow bowls and sprinkle with parsley and tarragon. Serve with bread for mopping up the sauce, or over noodles.

The Ultimate Hearty Minestrone

Grocery List

2 tablespoons butter

2 tablespoons olive oil

1 medium onion, diced (5 oz.)

2 stalks celery, sliced (5 oz.)

4 garlic cloves, minced (2 teaspoons)

2 cups green cabbage, chopped (12 oz.)

1 teaspoon salt

1/2 teaspoon freshly ground black pepper

8 cups vegetable stock or broth

3 large plum tomatoes, cored & chopped (12 oz.)

1 large russet potato, peeled & cut in 1/4" cubes (7 oz.)

15 ounces canned chickpeas, rinsed & drained

1 medium zucchini, cut in 1/4" cubes (7 oz.)

12 ounces fresh green beans, trimmed & cut in 1" pieces

2 large carrots, peeled & cut in 1/4 " pieces (9 oz.)

15 ounces canned kidney beans, rinsed & drained

8 large basil leaves, cut in thin strips

1/2 cup chopped fresh parsley

2 tablespoons chopped fresh oregano

1/2 cup parmesan cheese, freshly grated (1 1/2 oz.)

Instructions

Melt butter and olive oil in dutch oven or stock pot of at least 5 1/2 quart capacity. Set heat to medium and add onion, celery, garlic and cabbage. Mix Grocery List well; add salt and pepper. Saute' for about 10 minutes.

Once vegetables are translucent, add vegetable stock along with the tomatoes, potato and chickpeas. Bring to a boil then lower heat to medium and simmer for 30 minutes. Remove about 4 cups of mixture (mostly solids) to a heatproof container. Blend until smooth with an immersion blender. Return blended ingredients to pot to incorporate with soup. Alternately, a blender can be used for this process.

Add zucchini, green beans, carrots and kidney beans to pot and return to a boil. Reduce heat to medium-low and simmer for an additional 25 minutes.

Stir in the fresh herbs. Remove from heat and, if necessary, add salt and pepper to taste. Serve immediately, topped with freshly grated Parmesan cheese.

Hearty Tortellini and Spinach Soup

Grocery List

Olive oil

2 cloves garlic, minced

1 sweet onion, diced

1 roasted red pepper, diced

1 pound ground beef

6 cups chicken broth

1 24-ounce can San Marzano tomatoes

2 cups packed spinach

10 ounces fresh or frozen tortellini

Kosher salt + pepper to taste

Instructions

Heat a large soup pot over medium high heat. Add olive oil and heat. Add the garlic, onion and red pepper. Sauté until onion is softened.

Add ground beef and cook until browned and no longer pink.

Add chicken broth, San Marzano tomatoes, spinach and tortellini.

Bring to a boil and cook and until the tortellini is heated through. Taste for seasoning.

Sweet Corn Butter From Whitney Wright

Grocery List

8 ears fresh sweet corn, shucked

Butter and salt, to taste (optional)

Instructions

Cut off kernels: Use a chef's knife to cut the kernels from each ear. To wrangle the kernels, arrange towels around the cutting board and cut the corn in the center of the circle. Or balance the ear in the center of a Bundt pan and cut. Or lay the ear on its side and slice the kernels off with a sturdy chef's knife. 8 ears of corn will yield 4 to 5 cups of kernels. If you're a go-getter, you can also scrape the back of your knife along the cob to get the juice.

Blend (or juice): Your best move is to juice the kernels. But if you don't have a juicer, put the kernels in a blender or food processor and buzz them up like crazy—let the blender run on the highest speed (I'm talking the "liquefy" setting) for about 2 minutes. Once the kernels are blended into a smooth puree, pass the puree through a strainer with a rubber spatula. Ta-da! Corn juice.

Whisk and cook: Here's where the magic happens. Pour the juice into a medium saucepan. Heat the juice over medium heat, whisking constantly. Continue whisking until the mixture begins to thicken and the frothy bubbles begin to disappear, about 4 minutes. When the mixture is thick and bubbling, whisk and cook for about 30 seconds more. Remove from the heat.

Season (optional): Taste it—and look for sweet, smooth, earthy, and buttery. If you want, add a few pinches of salt and pats of butter. The corn butter will keep for about 3 to 5 days in the fridge.

Welsh Cawl

Grocery List

Stock

2-3 pounds boneless lamb shoulder (in one large piece) or lamb stew meat

Kosher salt and freshly ground black pepper

2 tablespoons extra virgin olive oil

1 large white or yellow onion, diced

2 large or 3 small shallots, diced

4 cups low-sodium vegetable stock

4 cups water

2 tablespoons (heaped) diced soup greens (or 1 small carrot, halved, and ½ bunch parsley)

Stew

3 large peeled Russet potatoes, sliced 1/2-inch thick

3 large carrots, sliced 1/2-inch thick

2 parsnips, peeled, sliced 1/2-inch thick

1 small celeriac bulb, peeled and diced, or 4 celery stalks, sliced 1/2-inch thick

Kosher salt and freshly ground black pepper

2 large or 3 small leeks (white and green parts), washed well and sliced 1/2-inch thick

Fresh parsley, roughly chopped, for serving

Hearty bread, for serving

Caerphilly (or English cheddar) cheese, for serving

Instructions

Season the meat all over with salt and pepper. Set aside.

In a large stockpot, sauté the onion and shallots in the olive oil over medium-high heat until they start to brown, 5-10 minutes. Add the meat and sauté for approximately 10 minutes.

Add stock and water, plus the diced soup greens (or carrot and parsley).

Bring to a rapid boil, then reduce heat and simmer for approximately one hour, or until the meat is tender and cooked through (registers at least 145°F with an instant-read thermometer). Remove the pot from the heat (removing and discarding carrot and celery). Transfer to a lidded container, or cover the pot and refrigerate for 8 hours, or overnight.

Use a spoon to skim the solidified fat from the surface of the stock and discard. Place the meat and stock in a large stock pot (or, if you chilled in the stock pot, simply place it back on the stove) with the peeled and sliced potatoes, carrots, parsnip, and celeriac.

Bring the mixture to a rapid boil over medium-high heat, then reduce heat to simmer for 15 minutes. Stir in the leeks, then continue to simmer for another 15 to 25 minutes, or until the vegetables are tender. If the stock seems to be drying out, add additional water.

Stir in the leeks during the last 15 minutes of simmering.

If using boneless lamb shoulder (or flank steak), remove the meat from the pot and slice to desired thickness.

Ladle the stew into bowls along with the sliced meat; if using stew meat, simply ladle into bowls. Top with parsley and serve with bread and cheese if desired.

The Cuban

Grocery List

The Cuban

4 good Cuban sandwich rolls (I posted a separate recipe for these here on food52.)

1 pound roasted and sliced Cuban Adobo Roasted Pork Shoulder (recipe is below)

4 - 6 generous slices good Swiss cheese

4 - 6 ounces finely sliced Black Forest or similar deli ham

Mayonnaise to taste

Four half-sour pickles, thinly sliced

Hearty brown mustard (I like a coarse mustard with horseradish)

Cuban Adobo Pork, Braise Roasted

1 3-pound pork shoulder

5 medium garlic cloves, peeled and mashed

2 teaspoons Kosher salt

1 ½ - 2 teaspoons freshly ground cumin seeds

2 tablespoons finely chopped fresh sage leaves

1 tablespoon finely chopped fresh oregano leaves

½ teaspoon freshly ground black pepper (I like Malabar) or white pepper

2 - 3 tablespoons olive oil

2 medium onions, peeled and thickly sliced

1 – 2 cups of chicken stock, heated

3 or 4 medium carrots, peeled and cut into bite-sized chunks (strictly optional, but nice to serve with the sauce)

Instructions

The Cuban

Heat panini press or other top and bottom grilling device for sandwiches.

Slice the rolls lengthwise and spread one side with mustard and the other side with mayonnaise.

Layer the ham, cheese, pork and pickles in whatever order you like. Press the two sides together.

Cook in the panini press until the grill lines are dark brown and sandwich is nice and warm.

Enjoy!! ;o)

Cuban Adobo Pork, Braise Roasted

Score the pork shoulder a few times about ¼ inch deep on each side.

Using a mortar and pestle, mash the garlic with the salt to make a paste. Add the cumin and sage leaves and pound a fe times to mix it into the garlic and salt. Add the pepper and the olive oil and stir to combine.

Rub the herb paste all over the pork should and into the crevices. Some people like to tie their pork shoulders up, but I generally don't, as I find you get more crispy bits that way. You certainly may, if you wish.

Put the roast in a bowl you can cover or a lidded glass storage container and refrigerate for at least six hours or, preferably, overnight. Bring the meat to room temperature for about an hour before roasting.

Preheat the oven the 375 degrees.

Put the onion slices in a braising pan or Dutch oven. Put the meat in on top of that. Cook for about 20 minutes, then add the stock. It should come up about ¼ of the way up the meat. If it doesn't, add a bit of water.

Cover and braise-roast for another hour, then turn the roast over. Add more stock or water if what you put in earlier has evaporated.

Cook for another half hour, then turn the roast over again and add more liquid if necessary. The onions will have released quite a bit, but depending on how much space there is on the bottom of the pan, it's not uncommon for the pan to dry out. Add the carrots now, if using.

Return the roast, uncovered, for yet another half hour, then check the meat with a fork. It should be very tender and should pull apart easily. At this point, I usually flip the roast over again and cook it for at least another 15 – 20 minutes. For pulled pork, you want the internal temperature to be at least 180 degrees. I think 190 is better - the hotter it is, the more collagen has broken down, making the meat really luscious.

Let the roast sit for at least 20 minutes after removing it, before slicing.

The onions can be pureed with the pan juices, and more stock if you like, using an immersion or other blender, to make a nice sauce for the roast.

Enjoy!!

Zurek (Polish Hangover Soup)

Grocery List

Zakwas

1/2 cup rye flour

2 garlic cloves, finely chopped

1 bay leaf

Soup

1/3 pound thick-cut smoked bacon, cut crosswise into 1/4-inch-wide pieces

2 medium onions, coarsely chopped

2 1/2 pounds kielbasa or bratwurst, cut into 1/2-inch-thick slices

1 large carrot, halved lengthwise and cut into 3/4-inch-thick slices

1 large parsnip, quartered lengthwise and cut into 3/4-inch-thick slices

1 medium celery root, peeled and cut into 1/2-inch cubes

8 sprigs fresh flat-leaf parsley, plus finely chopped fresh parsley for garnish

3 fresh or dried bay leaves

2 teaspoons dried marjoram

1/8 teaspoon ground allspice

Kosher salt

1/4 cup drained prepared horseradish

1/4 teaspoon freshly ground white pepper

Sour cream, for garnish

3 or 4 hard-boiled eggs, peeled and halved, for garnish

2 cups coarsely chopped dill pickles (about 4 medium), for garnish

Chopped fresh dill, for garnish

Instructions

Zakwas

For the zakwas: Pour 2 cups boiling water into a heatproof 1-quart jar or glass bowl. Let cool to warm.

Stir the flour, garlic, and bay leaf into the warm water. Tightly cover/seal the jar or bowl with plastic wrap (use a rubber band or two to hold the wrap tightly) and let sit in a warm, dark place (like a cupboard) for 4 to 5 days; "burp" the mixture every 2 days by removing the plastic wrap to let the air out, then resealing it again (this will prevent a little culinary explosion). Alternatively, you can seal the jar or bowl with cheesecloth (more breathable), held tightly with a rubber band, and you will not have to burp the mixture.

The zakwas is ready when it has a pungent fragrance, a solid, spongy deposit on top, and a light brown-gray liquid at the bottom. Scrape off any green or moldy bits that appear on the top (a healthy sign of the fermentation process and not dangerous!), and remove and discard the bay leaf. Strain the zakwas through a sieve into a bowl; discard the solids. You'll have about 1½ cups liquid. Use however much you have; the exact amount is not important.

Soup

For the soup: In a large Dutch oven or other wide heavy pot, cook the bacon over medium-high heat, stirring occasionally, until golden and crisp, 5 to 7 minutes. Using a slotted spoon, transfer to a medium bowl. Add the onions to the pot and cook, stirring occasionally, until tender and lightly golden, 12 to 14 minutes. Transfer to the bowl with the bacon. Add the kielbasa or bratwurst to the pot and cook, stirring occasionally, until golden brown, 12 to 15 minutes. Transfer to the onion mixture. Pour off and discard the fat from the pot.

Add the carrot, parsnip, celery root, parsley sprigs, bay leaves, marjoram, allspice, 1 teaspoon salt, and 7 cups water to the pot, bring to a simmer, and cook until the vegetables are almost tender but with a little bite, 12 to 15 minutes.

Add the zakwas, horseradish, and onion mixture to the pot, return the soup to a simmer, and cook until the vegetables are tender and the broth is flavorful, 10 to 12 minutes. Stir in the white pepper. Season to taste with salt. Remove and discard the parsley sprigs and bay leaves.

Spoon the soup into bowls. Top each bowl with a big dollop of sour cream, a hard-boiled egg half, the chopped pickles, and some dill or parsley, and serve.

Italian Wedding Soup With Parm Broth

Grocery List

Parm Broth:

1 pound Parmesan rinds

1 yellow onion, halved, skin left on

1 head garlic, halved crosswise

6 sprigs flat-leaf parsley

1/2 teaspoon black peppercorns

3/4 teaspoon kosher salt

Meatballs:

2/3 cup panko

3 tablespoons whole milk

1/2 pound ground beef

1/2 pound ground pork or sweet Italian sausage, casing removed

1 large egg

1/4 cup grated Parmesan

1/4 cup chopped flat-leaf parsley

2 garlic cloves, minced

1/2 teaspoon red pepper flakes

1/2 teaspoon ground fennel

Soup:

3 tablespoons extra-virgin olive oil

1 or 2 carrots, medium dice (about 1/2 cup total)

1 or 2 celery stalks, medium dice (about 1/2 cup total)

1 small fennel bulb, thinly sliced

2 garlic cloves, minced

Kosher salt and freshly ground black pepper

6 cups torn hearty greens, such as escarole or other chicories

To serve: chopped flat-leaf parsley, lemon wedges, grated Parmesan, and red pepper flakes (optional)

Instructions

Make the Parm broth: Add all the ingredients to a stockpot, along with 12 cups of water. Bring to a simmer and cook uncovered for 2 to 2 1/2 hours, stirring occasionally to keep the cheese from sticking to the bottom of the pot. When ready, the broth should look cloudy and have a deep Parmesan flavor. Strain the broth into a clean, heatproof bowl or pot, pressing on the solids to extract as much liquid as possible. Taste and add more salt and pepper if needed. I like a lot of pepper in this broth.

Meanwhile, while the broth is simmering, work on the meatballs: Combine panko and milk in a medium mixing bowl and stir. Let sit for a few minutes to let the bread crumbs absorb the liquid—this will give our meatballs moisture and a lighter texture. Add the beef, pork or sausage, and egg to the panko. Toss lightly to combine, followed by the Parmesan, parsley, garlic, pepper flakes, and ground fennel. Mix with clean hands to combine, but try not to overwork the mixture.

To finish the soup, Add the olive oil to a stockpot set over medium heat. Add the carrots, celery, fennel, garlic, and a healthy pinch of salt. Let vegetables sweat until they just begin to take on color. Add all the greens at once and give them a stir to wilt down. Add all of the Parmesan broth and bring to a high simmer. Using a tablespoon measure or two large soup spoons (one to scoop, one to scrape off), scoop the meatball mixture and gently plop into the simmering broth. Repeat until all the mixture has been used up. Let the soup gently bubble, lowering the heat if needed, till the meatballs begin to float and are cooked through, 10 to 15 minutes. Taste the broth and season with salt and pepper as needed.

Serve with chopped parsley, a squeeze of lemon juice, and grated Parmesan if desired. Or, my personal favorite, red pepper flakes.

Quinoa & Roasted Sweet Potato Superfood Salad

Grocery List

salad

1/2 cup quinoa

1 sweet potato

1/3 cup walnuts or pumpkin seeds

1 avocado

3 cups hearty mixed greens

2 pinches salt and pepper

chili lime vinaigrette

1 lime juiced

1/2 cup olive oil

1/2 teaspoon chili powder

1 teaspoon honey

Instructions

Prepare quinoa per package instructions.

Preheat oven to 350. Peel your sweet potato and cut into 1-inch chunks. Toss the sweet potato with olive oil and salt and pepper. Place on parchment-lined cookie sheet and roast for about 25 minutes, flipping them over once in the middle of roasting.

Slice avocado.

Prepare the dressing. Then combine the warm ingredients (quinoa and sweet potato) and add half of your dressing to those ingredients.

Toss the remaining ingredients with the dressing and compose your salad.

Oma's Chicken Paprikash

Grocery List

Paprikash

2 tablespoons vegetable oil

1 large onion, diced

4 tablespoons sweet Hungarian paprika, heaping

2 chicken breasts, quartered (or 4 bone-in thighs)

2 cups water

1/2 cup sour cream

1 tablespoon flour

1 pinch salt and pepper, to taste

Dumplings

3 eggs

1 teaspoon vegetable oil

3/4 cup water

3 cups flour

Instructions

In a large pot or Dutch oven, heat oil, and add onion. Cook, stirring occasionally, until almost translucent. Add paprika it will seem like a lot, but trust me, the more the better and stir to combine. Heat through for several more adding the paprika at the beginning of the cooking process intensifies the smoky-sweet, robust flavor and cook until the onions are cooked through, stirring almost continuously.

Add chicken and stir to coat with paprika, let it brown slightly, and add 2 cups of water. Bring to a boil, then turn heat down and simmer for 45 minutes to an hour. Add more water if needed.

Meanwhile, make the dumplings. Combine all dumpling Grocery List in the bowl of your stand mixer. Mix with bread hook until combined the dough will be thick and sticky. In a pot of boiling, salted water, drop in 5 tablespoon-sized dollops at a time, and cook for 1 to 2 minutes, until cooked through. The dumplings should be slippery on the outside, and bready on the inside. Set aside a bowlfull for the next day's breakfast, and refrigerate it overnight.

Before serving, add the remaining dumplings to paprikash.

In a small bowl, whisk together sour cream, a spoonful of flour, and a splash of water, and stir into the paprikash. Add salt and pepper to taste. Give the chicken a rough shred with your fork, and serve in a bowl, as you would a stew.

The next morning, slice the dumplings you set aside, and heat with a healthy-sized pat of butter. Top with a good shower of cinnamon and sugar.

DESSERTS

Pudding & Custard

Grocery List

For the pudding:

50 grams plain wholemeal flour

1 piece egg

75 milliliters unsweetened almond milk

1 tablespoon coconut oil

For the custard:

600 milliliters coconut milk

3 tablespoons honey or maple syrup

1 piece vanilla pod

9 pieces egg yolks

Instructions

Preheat the oven to 200C/390F.

Add coconut oil to the bottom of each muffin tin, then heat for 5 mins in the oven.

Meanwhile, beat all the egg yolks for the custard in a bowl.

Add the milk, honey/maple syrup and vanilla for the custard to a saucepan and heat gently over a medium heat until warm, but not boiling.

Whisk the egg and flour for the puddings together and then slowly add the milk, add the mixture to the muffin tins and place in the oven for 10 minutes.

Add the beaten egg yolks to the custard pan and stir continuously until everything is combined, then turn down to a low heat for another 15 minutes until thickened, whisking occasionally.

Once everything is ready serve with fresh fruit, cinnamon and healthy jam.

Pears En Pillowette with Almond Mascarpone Cream

Grocery List

Poached Pear Pacckets

6 14" Parchment Paper Circles

4-6 Ripe but slightly firm, medium Bartlett or Red Bartlett Pears

3 - 4 tablespoons Sugar

~OR~

2-3 tablespoons Light Agave Nectar

6 teaspoons Unsalted Butter, Room Temp.

3 teaspoons Fresh Grated Ginger

Pinch Fresh Ground Black Pepper

Pinch Loose Red Chai or any Quality Red Tea

Dash Lemon Juice

Almond Mascarpone Cream

16 ounces Heavy Whipping Cream

8 ounces Mascarpone Cheese

1.5 tablespoons Light Agave Nectar

1/4 teaspoon Pure Almond Extract or Almond Liquor

Instructions

Preheat your oven to bake at 425F and start cutting out your 14" parchment circles. I used a pie crust protector or a large plate for mine. Just be sure to cut them large enough or the packets wont seal properly when cooking.

Make your cream first to save time, mess and counter space later. Combine mascarpone cheese, heavy cream, and sugar then whisk until it just begins to thicken. Add almond flavor and whisk until it reaches a firm peak state. Contact cover with wrap and set aside in the fridge.

Next, prepare your Grocery List for the pear packets: Take butter out of the fridge, grate ginger, grind pepper, and measure out sugar and tea. Place your flavor ingredients in pinch bowls or the equivalent for easy access.

Wash and slice your pears length wise then remove the cores with either a spoon or even better with a melon baller. Slice them, skin on, into about domino sized pieces. The thicker, the firmer here but dont go much thicker than 1/4" or thinner than 1/8"... I like to do this step as needed and just before assembly so the enzymes in the pears don't have a chance to brown the flesh when exposed to oxygen in the air

Time to start your assembly! Place about 1/2 to 3/4 of a pear in a little stack in the center of your parchment circle. Add a pinch of pepper, pinch or tea, sugar or agave to , small dash of lemon juice then top with 1/2 teaspoon ginger and lastly with 1 healthy teaspoon butter. Take the edges of the parchment circle in 4 places, bring them together and twist to seal. Be sure to get a good, tight twist on these little packets so steam cant escape too readily while baking.

Place the packets in a shallow sheet pan and bake 10 - 14 minutes until the twisted tops of the parchment start to turn brown. Remove from heat and serve stil wrapped packets in small bowls along with small cups of cream. I like to serve the cream in espresso cups or small teacups for some extra flare. Enjoy!

Tang Yuan (Glutinous Rice Balls)

Grocery List

Ginger Syrup:

1 cup (213 grams) light brown sugar

1 (3-inch) piece ginger (about 40 grams), sliced

Filling & Dough:

1/2 cup (50 grams) packed toasted black sesame powder

3 tablespoons (48 grams) tahini or black sesame paste

1 tablespoon plus 1½ teaspoons granulated sugar

1 pinch kosher salt

1 1/2 cups (275 grams) Mochiko sweet rice flour

3/4 cup (177 milliliters) boiling water, plus more as needed

Instructions

Ginger Syrup:

In a small pot, bring 6 cups of water to a boil. Add the brown sugar, whisking to dissolve, then add the ginger. Reduce the heat to medium-low, bring to a very low simmer, and cover the pot. Let simmer while you make the dumplings.

Filling & Dough:

In a food processor, pulse the sesame powder with the sugar and salt until finely ground. Add the tahini and pulse just until it comes together. Transfer to a small bowl, cover with a damp towel, and set aside.

Place the flour in a medium bowl. Pour the boiling water over and incorporate with a rubber spatula. Let cool slightly. Knead the dough with your hands—it will look and feel dry at first, but keep kneading until it comes together. Form a smooth ball, return to the bowl, and cover with a damp towel. This dough dries out very quickly, and while you can revive it by massaging it with a bit more water, it's best to work fast and keep it covered with a damp cloth or paper towel at all times.

Portion out the dough into 30-gram pieces. Roll each into a ball, return to the bowl, and cover again with the damp towel. Keep a bowl of water to dip your hands into and a damp towel next to you while you work.

Working one at a time to prevent the dough from drying out, gently press the dough to flatten into a circle around 3 inches wide. If the dough feels dry or stiff, dip your hands into the bowl of water and massage the dough until it feels hydrated again.

Using a 1-teaspoon measuring spoon, scoop some of the sesame filling into the center of the dough, then gently pull the sides together to enclose. Roll into a ball (just as you'd roll a Parker House Roll) and set aside. Repeat with the remaining filling and dough.

Bring the ginger syrup to a healthy simmer, then gently plop the dumplings in one at a time. Cook for about 10 minutes, until they float and the dough looks slightly translucent. The filling should be hot (cut one open to see).

Spoon some syrup into 2 or 3 bowls, along with the dumplings. Leave the ginger behind in the pot. Serve hot.

Do Ahead: Once formed, the dumplings can be frozen for up to 3 months. To freeze, arrange them flat on a sheet tray. Once frozen, store in a zip-top bag or airtight container. Any extra filling can be refrigerated for up to 2 weeks or frozen for up to 3 months. I do not recommend keeping the tang yuan in the fridge after you've cooked them. The cooked dough becomes a firmer and even unpleasant texture when reheated.

Raspberry-Lime Parfaits with Whipped Goat Cheese

Grocery List

2 avocados

2 limes

2-4 tablespoons Honey

1 package goat cheese, softened

2 tablespoons water

1 pint fresh raspberries

Instructions

1. Put the juice of two fresh limes, the flesh of two whole avocados, and 2 to 4 tablespoons of fresh, local honey into a food processor. Blend until smooth. The puree can be as sweet as the palate of

the person making it desires. We use about two tablespoons.

Put the package of goat cheese, along with at least two tablespoons of water into the stand mixer. The water is also approximate. Blend with the whisk attachment until the goat cheese is soft and smooth. The water is just enough to make it thinner, a similar consistency to the avocado-lime puree. Thicker than pancake batter but not as thick as muffin batter.

Compose the parfaits in a clear glass. Add a hearty scoop of the lime/avocado puree, a layer of raspberries, a healthy scoop of goat cheese, a layer of raspberries and repeat until the parfaits are full. Add many raspberries as they are the star of the dish, and the goat cheese's strong flavor and lime puree just enhance the berries.

Huckleberry Yogurt Pseudo Trifle

Grocery List

2 pieces Hearty Whole Grain Bread or Baguette Thick Sliced

1 handful Cherries

1 handful Red Huckleberries (or another berry of your choice)

6 tablespoons Greek Vanilla Yogurt

1 tablespoon Peanut butter (optional)

2 teaspoons Grand Marnier (optional)

1 handful Strawberries

Instructions

Toast thickly sliced whole grain bread or baguette until golden. Break off bite-sized chunks and place them into a serving bowl.

Throw in a third of your huckleberries, cherries, and mint (shredded). Drizzle in a teaspoon of honey and grand marnier (optional). Top with just enough yogurt to cover the bread.

Repeat step 1 and 2 for the second layer. For added flavour, coat the second slice of bread in peanut butter before tearing off chunks into the bowl.

To finish, add the remaining ingredients with some sliced strawberry. Place covered in the fridge for 30 minutes and serve.

Darjeeling Tea Pain Perdu with Condensed Milk Butter

Grocery List

For the condensed milk butter

4 ounces sweet (unsalted) butter, softened

1 can sweetened condensed milk

1/4 cup powdered sugar

2 teaspoons flaky salt

For the Darjeeling tea pain perdu

4 1-inch thick slices day old brioche

1 1/2 cups heavy cream

4 bags Darjeeling tea, or 4 tablespoons tea leaves

1 split vanilla bean

2 tablespoons honey

4 eggs

1 pinch salt

1/4 cup raw sugar

3 tablespoons clarified butter or ghee

Instructions

For the condensed milk butter

Beat butter and sugar with a hand mixer or in the bowl of a standing mixer on high, until creamy and light.

With mixer running, slowly pour in condensed milk to incorporate.

Turn off mixer and fold in salt.

The butter will keep for a few days in the fridge.

For the Darjeeling tea pain perdu

Combine cream, vanilla bean, tea, and honey in a saucepan.

Bring to a boil over medium heat, then reduce heat and let simmer 4 to 5 minutes. Remove from heat and let sit at least 1 hour. Strain and cool. (You can do this a day ahead.)

Whisk eggs with salt. Whisk cooled cream into eggs slowly.

Dip bread into cream/egg mixture and set in baking dish, letting everything soak in well.

Pour remaining cream/egg mixture over top and let sit for at least an hour or refrigerate overnight.

Heat butter in a saute pan over medium high heat.

Sprinkle bread with raw sugar. Fry first on the non-sugared side, then flip, making sure to cook all the way through.

Serve warm with a healthy dollop of condensed milk butter.

Chili Chocolate Mousse Cake

Grocery List

13 ounces , or 370 grams, chili-infused chocolate (or another dark chocolate of your taste)

6 ounces , or 170 grams, butter, plus more for greasing the pan

8 eggs, separated

1/2 cup , or 90 grams, light brown sugar

1/3 cup , or 65 grams, white sugar

2 tablespoons vanilla sugar (or 1 tsp vanilla extract)

Instructions

Pre-heat oven to 175 C/350 F. Butter a spring-form pan, both the bottom and sides. Line the bottom of the pan with parchment paper and butter the top of the parchment paper.

Melt the chocolate and butter in a bain-marie/double boiler, stirring to blend. Once melted and mixed, let cool.

Meanwhile, separate the eggs. Beat the egg yolks and sugars (including the vanilla sugar if you have it) until the mixture is very thick, pale, and creamy. If using vanilla extract, mix it in.

Add the cooled chocolate and butter mixture to the egg yolk and sugar mixture. Mix until blended.

In a separate bowl, whisk the egg whites until stiff peaks form. Add a healthy dollop of the egg white to the chocolate mixture from step 4. Fold vigorously... don't worry about deflating the egg whites. Once incorporated, add 1/4 of the remaining egg whites and fold to incorporate. Now is the time to worry about deflating the egg whites! Once incorporated, add another 1/4 of the egg whites and fold. Continue until you have incorporated all of the egg whites.

You should now have a lovely chocolate mousse! Pour half of the mousse into your prepared spring-form pan. Bake, uncovered, for 20 minutes. Keep the other half of the mousse in the mixing bowl on your counter.

After the 20 minutes of baking, remove the mousse from the oven. Pour the remaining (uncooked) mousse into the now baked mousse. If the spring-form looks like it will overflow, wait a few minutes for the cake to deflate, then pour in the rest of the mousse. Allow the pan to come to room temperature, then freeze the cake for 2-12 hours. After a maximum of 12 hours, remove the cake from the freezer and keep in the refrigerator until ready to serve.

Pumpkin Pots de Creme with Orange Cranberry Whipped Cream

Grocery List

Pumpkin Pots de Creme

1 1/2 cups heavy cream

2/3 cup pumpkin puree

1/2 cup maple syrup

8 egg yolks

1/2 teaspoon cinnamon

1/4 teaspoon nutmeg

1/8 teaspoon clove

1 cup ginger cookie pieces

1 pinch salt

Orange Cranberry Whipped Cream

1 cup heavy cream

2/3 cup fresh cranberries

3 tablespoons maple syrup

1/4 teaspoon orange extract

Instructions

In a large bowl whisk together egg yolks and salt until yolks lighten in color. Set aside.

In a sauce pot, stir to combine cream, pumpkin, spices and maple syrup and heat until just simmering. Remove from heat.

Slowly pour the cream/pumpkin mixture into the yolks while rapidly whisking to combine.

Divide the ginger cookie pieces among 8 ramekin containers. Pour the pumpkin creme mixture over the ginger cookies, until evenly divided.

Place ramekins on a deep baking pan on the middle rack of a 375 F degree preheated oven. Pour hot water into the baking pan until it reaches just under half way up the sides of the ramekin dishes. Bake for 35 minutes. Remove the dishes from the water bath and set aside to cool. Refrigerate for at least 2 hours before serving.

To make the whipped cream: Combine cream, maple syrup, and orange extract in a large mixing bowl. Whisk by hand or with mixer until soft peaks can easily maintain shape. In a food processor or blender, pulse the fresh cranberries as finely as possible, then fold this into the whipped cream until fully combined.

When you are ready to serve, remove the ramekins from the fridge, add a healthy swirl of whipped cream and enjoy!

Dark Chocolate Bark

Grocery List

1 pound good quality dark chocolate (70% or higher) like a Ghirardelli or Scharfenberger

1/2 cup Goji berries

1/2 cup pumpkin seeds

1/2 unsweetened coconut flakes

Instructions

Chop chocolate. Place in a bowl over simmering water. DO NOT allow the bottom the bowl to touch the water (the heat from the water will burn the chocolate.

While chocolate is melting prepare a sheet pan with parchment paper.

When chocolate begins to melt turn heat off and stir the chocolate with a spatula until completely melted. Pour onto prepared sheet pan and smooth out to desired thickness - about 1/8 inch thick.

Place in the refrigerator for at least 15 minutes to set. Feel free to add any toppings that you want. We just liked this combination! You can also make this with milk chocolate or white chocolate or even a mix/swirl (look for our white chocolate bark coming soon). We like the flavonoids and the health benefits of dark chocolate

Roasted Peaches and Yogurt

Grocery List

2 Peaches

1 Yogurt/Something Creamy

White Wine

Nutmeg

Cinnamon

2-3 tablespoons Butter

1 splash Lime Juice

Tablespoon Raw Honey

Instructions

Slice/Core peaches into slices

Warm your pan of choice with butter and honey – I used a fairly low heat so make sure the honey didn't burn.

Place the peaches in your pan and thoroughly coat them with the butter and honey mixture

Pour in a dash... or more of your wine wine, and toss on whatever toppings are your favorite. My personal favorites are nutmeg, cinnamon and some lime juice for a sassy splash – THEN: Turn down the heat and simmer, covering the top of the pan to insure you get those flavors.

While that's slowly simmering, preheat your oven to around 200C and whip up whatever sweet creamy yogurt you have. My strategy for this meal was to be somewhat healthy, so I used Fage 0% Yogurt and whipped it into a delicious center of my plate. Obviously the option to just having heavy whipping cream or even better… ice cream is open to you.

After 7-8 minutes of simmer, throw the peaches and the pan into the oven for 10ish minutes

Take out the peaches let them cool, but only for a little bit – because that mixture of sweet creamy goodness and warm soul-warming heaven can only last for a brief moment.

Intense Strawberry Coconut Ice Cream + Almond Waffle Cone

Grocery List

Intense Strawberry Coconut Ice Cream - custard based & dairy free

6 egg yolks

3 cans of full fat coconut milk

1/2 cup sugar

1 tablespoon potato starch

2 cups strawberries, washed & halved

zest of 6 lemons

Almond Waffle Cones & Bowls - gluten free

2/3 cup almond flour

1/4 teaspoon salt

2 eggs

2 tablespoons honey

2 tablespoons coconut oil, melted

Instructions

Intense Strawberry Coconut Ice Cream - custard based & dairy free

for the strawberries, vitamix them until smooth as possible. it'll equal out to about 1 1/2 cups liquid. reduce down in small saucepan on low heat, throwing a few healthy sprinkles of lemon zest. you're aiming to get as much liquid/moisture out of the mixture as possible, leaving behind a thick sauce. i reduced it down to about 1/2 cup – 3/4 cup — basically until i got tired of babysitting it.

for the ice cream base, it's my usual egg custard base. in a medium saucepan add in 2 1/2 cans of coconut milk, reserving the remaining for later. heat up the milk with the sugar until fully incorporated. add in a few healthy sprinkles of lemon zest. in a small bowl, separate your eggs. whisk the yolks, and then with a ladle pour in the hot coconut milk all the while whisking the yolks. this is tempering the yolks so it doesn't scramble. if you want, add in another ladle-full. then slowly add in the warmed through yolk mixture into the saucepan, still whisking. you want the mixture to be fully incorporated. keep the heat on medium and keeping mixing until the mixture has thickened, about 10-15 minutes. at this point, with the remaining half can of coconut milk stir in the potato starch, then add mixture to the custard. this will thicken the custard even more, while also preventing full on ice crystals from forming when the ice cream is in the freezer.

remove custard from saucepan and allow cool. cover and refrigerate for a few hours, ideally overnight. same thing with the strawberry sauce.

when ready, pour custard base into ice maker and churn, then add in the strawberry sauce. churn according to manufacturer's specs.

*note – technically, you could mix the strawberry sauce and custard before adding to the machine but it seemed like a whole lot of mixing and we figured the machine was well capable of doing that step for us. we opted to pour the custard first because there's a lot more of it than the sauce, and there's always a thin layer of ice cream along the edge of the canister that is difficult to scrape out when frozen. we figured we could "waste" that layer of mainly custard rather than of the strawberry sauce.

Almond Waffle Cones & Bowls - gluten free

in a vitamix, blitz everything until smooth

heat your waffle cone maker to #3. pour batter into it, aim for 1/4 cup (let's be smart, eyeball it and try not to get greedy) and cook for about 2-3 minutes. check on it after 1 minute, aim for a nice golden brown shade. very quickly and carefully peel the waffle out with a small spatula and shape over a bowl or cup, or into a cone. allow to cool.

a trick: i added a few chocolate chips in the bottom of the cone, the residual warm of the cooking melted it a bit and it created a stopper. if you're a slow ice cream eater, like dw, hopefully no leaks!

No-Bake Berries & Cream Cake

Grocery List

Lemon-Honey Syrup

1/3 cup water

2 tablespoons raw honey

1 lemon, zest and juice

10 basil leaves

The Cake

1/4 cup water

1 cup blueberry preserves

1 1/4 cups blueberries

3/4 cup black raspberries

8 ounces Neufchâtel cheese, softened

1/4 cup confectioners sugar

1 teaspoon vanilla extract

1 cup heavy cream

a few basil leaves, minced

1 loaf of pound cake (approx. 9" x 4" x 4"), cut into 1/3-inch slices

lemon-honey syrup

Instructions

Combine the water, honey, and lemon zest in a small sauce pan. Heat until the honey has completely dissolved into the water, then remove from heat. Muddle the basil and add it to the pan. Let sit for 20 minutes, then strain and stir in the lemon juice.

Combine the water, berries, and preserves in a sauce pan. Cook over medium heat until it begins to thicken (approximately 15 minutes). Remove from heat and let cool.

Beat together the Neufchâtel, confectioners sugar, and vanilla. In a separate bowl, whip the heavy cream to stiff peaks, then fold in the Neufchâtel mixture.

Arrange pound cake slices on the bottom of a 9-inch springform pan, cutting to fill in gaps where needed. Brush the pound cake layer with a healthy amount of the lemon-honey syrup. Spread half of the berry mixture on top of the pound cake and sprinkle with minced basil. Spread half of the whipped cream over top of the berry layer. Repeat with another layer of pound cake, lemon-honey syrup, remaining berry mixture, basil, and the rest of the whipped cream.

Cover cake with plastic wrap and refrigerate for at least 5 hours, or overnight. When ready to serve, run a knife around the inner edge of the pan. Release from the pan and top with fresh berries.

Gingerbread Porter Cake with Cacao Nibs

Grocery List

10 tablespoons salted butter

1 cup dark molasses

1 cup dark brown sugar, packed

1 cup dark porter beer

2 cups cake flour

2 teaspoons baking soda

Dash salt

2 teaspoons unsweetened cocoa powder

2 teaspoons ground ginger

2 teaspoons ground cinnamon

1/4 teaspoon ground cloves

1 cup sour cream

2 eggs, beaten

1/3 + cups raw cacao nibs*

Instructions

Preheat oven to 325 degrees. Butter and flour a 10 inch springform pan. In a large saucepan over medium heat, melt the butter. Stir in the molasses, brown sugar and beer and heat until sugar is melted and mixture is smooth. In a separate bowl, whisk together the cake flour, baking soda, salt, cocoa powder, ginger, cinnamon and cloves.

Pour the melted butter and molasses mixture into the dry mixture and whisk until smooth. Whisk in the sour cream and then whisk in the eggs. Fold in 1/3 cup of the raw cacao nibs. Pour the batter into the prepared springform pan and sprinkle remaining 3 tablespoons cacao nibs on top. Bake for approximately 1 hour, or until toothpick inserted into center comes out clean. Cool, then unmold.

Raw cacao nibs are made from organic cacao beans that have been peeled and chopped. They're not sweet, but have an intense cocoa flavor with a tiny hint of bitterness (in a good way). They're addictive. Luckily, they're also really healthy for you- considered a superfood high in iron, fiber and antioxidents.

Fig & Cardamom Spiced Tiramisu

Grocery List

Filling

1 cup dried figs

4 tablespoons reserved liquid from soaking dried figs (see Instructions Step 1)

1 teaspoon vanilla extract

1 pound mascarpone cheese (2 8-ounce containers)

1 tablespoon ground cardamom (plus a few dashes reserved for finishing)

1 teaspoon ground cinnamon

1 cup heavy cream

3/4 cup confectioners/powdered sugar

Soak, Cookies and Topping

1/2 cup fresh-brewed espresso or strong coffee

1/2 cup sugar

1/2 cup heavy cream

36-40 pieces ladyfingers aka savoiardi (hard cookie version, not soft)

1-2 ounces excellent quality dark/bittersweet chocolate

Whipped cream (optional)

Instructions

As much as 24 hours prior to making tiramisu place dried figs in a heat proof container (a jar works fine). Pour boiling or very hot water over and soak for at least one hour until puffed up and rehydrated. If soaking overnight: cover and refrigerate.

Chopped soaked figs into quarters and blend in a food processor with 4 tablespoons of the liquid reserved from soaking.

For the filling: Combine pulverized figs, vanilla extract, mascarpone cheese, ground cardamom, ground cinnamon, heavy cream and confectioners sugar in a medium-large bowl. Combine well then beat (with a whisk by hand or with a blender) until stiffened - to a soft peak.

In a separate bowl: combine espresso (while hot) with heavy cream and sugar for the soak. Stir well to dissolve sugar.

Working in small batches quickly toss ladyfinger cookies in the soaking liquid. The cookies do not need to become softened or else they will quickly fall apart - simply place in the soak, roll over and then place into the bottom or a trifle or baking dish. Line the entire bottom of you dish with soaked cookies.

If you are working with a larger dish spread half of the filling over the cookies. If working with a smaller dish or trifle container, use a third of your filling.

Place another layer of soaked ladyfinger cookies over the filling. Again, spread filling over cookies. Repeat layering until complete.

Finish with a final layer of cream filling, a hearty helping of shredded chocolate*, an a few dashes of ground cardamom. To shred chocolate if it is in a bar form: Can be accomplished with a grater, microplaner, or even a potato peeler. Optional but recommended: Add a layer of whipped cream before shredded chocolate & cardamom. Fresh whipped is preferred (whip 1 cup cream until stiffened, add a tablespoon or so of confectioners sugar until sweetened to your taste)

Chill thoroughly and enjoy!

SNACKS

Balilah with Preserved Lemons and Pomegranates

Grocery List

1 cup dried chickpeas, soaked overnight

1 1/2 cups pomegrante arils

1 preserved lemon

2 shallots or 1 medium-large red onion, finely diced

1 tablespoon ground, toasted cumin seeds

Kosher salt to taste

1 cup packed finely chopped parsely

1 optional green serrano chile, deseeded and finely chopped

1/2 teaspoon fresh cracked peppercorn

2 tablespoons extra virgin olive oil

1 pinch baking soda

Instructions

Rinse the plumped up chickpeas and cover with enough water in a large pot. Add a pinch of baking soda and bring to boil. Cover and simmer for about 45 minutes until the chickpeas are soft but not mushy. Rinse the cooked beans, drain and set aside to cool to room temperature.

Remove and discard the seeds from the preserved lemon. Chop the fruit finely and using the flat surface of the knife, crush the pulp to mush (peel, pulp & juice). Transfer the entire lemon mush into a mixing bowl. Combine with the olive oil, cumin, chile (adjust as per your personal heat preference or omit), peppercorn, onions and parsley.

Add the chickpeas and the pomegranate arils to the preserved lemon mixture and gently fold to coat the chickpeas. Taste for seasoning and adjust for salt. (The preserved lemon already is quite salty, so add the salt carefully). Serve as an appetizer or as a healthy lunchtime salad served on a large lettuce leaf 'bowl'.

Bar Pizza-It's What You Crave

Grocery List

2 teaspoons extra-virgin olive oil

1 traditional 10-inch flour tortilla

2-3 tablespoons pizza sauce, homemade ot otherwise

mozzarella cheese, both fresh and grated

1 Fresno pepper, thinly sliced

flat leaf parsley, minced

Instructions

Place the top rack approximately 7 to 8-inches from the broiler. Heat the broiler.

Organize all you ingredients and place them within arms reach from the stove.

Place a 12-inch cast iron skillet over medium high heat. Add olive oil and swirl the pan to coat the entire bottom surface. The oil should be very hot. Place the tortilla into the pan and brown it deeply. Turn the tortilla.

Leave the tortilla in the pan while you sauce it. Place a healthy dollop of pizza sauce into the middle of the tortilla. Using a spoon spiral the sauce outward. If you don't have enough sauce dollop on a small amount and continue spreading.

Sprinkle the pizza with grated mozzarella, spread out the pepperoni evenly, and top with torn pieces of fresh mozzarella.

Place the skillet into the oven. Turn on the oven light and keep and eye on the pizza. It will melt quickly and begin to brown just as fast. When it is bubbling and brown, using an oven mit, remove it from the oven. Tilt the pan at about a 45 degree angle and using the tongs, pinch the very edge closest to the cutting board and gently slide the pizza out and onto the board. Sprinkle with parsley and pepper, slice and serve.

Broccoli Rabe & Fresh Mozzarella Panini

Grocery List

1/2 a bunch of fresh broccoli rabe, chopped into thirds

4 flat anchovies packed in oil, finely chopped

4-6 garlic cloves, sliced thin

1 tablespoon extra-virgin olive oil

pinch of salt

2 wedges ciabetta bread (or other hearty bread), sliced in half

4 thin slices fresh mozzarella

harissa

Instructions

Quickly steam (or blanch) the broccoli rabe until it is just crisp tender and set aside.

Cook the anchovies and garlic in olive oil until the garlic just begins to turn golden and the anchovies begin to dissolve, about 2-3 minutes. Add the broccoli rabe to the pan, sprinkle it with a pinch of salt and cook (stirring frequently) an additional 3-4 minutes.

Heat a panini or sandwich press according to manufacturer's instructions until hot. Brush one side of the bread slices with olive oil and place on a work surface. Layer the broccoli rabe mixture and two slices of mozzarella on each bottom slice. Spread the top slice with harissa and place on the sandwich.

Put sandwiches on the press, pull down the top and cook until the cheese has melted and the ciabatta is browned and crisp, 4 to 7 minutes.

Spring Toast

Grocery List

Pea Hummus

2 cups cooked sweet peas

1 tablespoon tahini

2 cloves garlic

1 tablespoon olive oil

juice half of one lemon

1 pinch sea salt

1 handful cilantro and/or mint

Spring Toast

2-3 tablespoons pea hummus, recipe above

1 piece hearty gluten-free toast

1/2 avocado, sliced

1/4 cup sprouts of choice

1 pinch sea salt

1 dash good quality olive oil

Instructions

Pea Hummus

Place all ingredients in food processor. Blend until smooth.

Taste for seasoning and adjust as necessary.

Place in sealed container. Store covered in refrigerator for 2-3 days.

Spring Toast

Toast bread.

Smear pea hummus over toast, then place sliced avocado on top.

Sprinkle with sprouts and sea salt. Drizzle with olive oil and eat immediately.

Roman Zucchini Fritters with Parmigiano Cheese

Grocery List

1 cup or so of semolina flour

3/4 cup or so of fresh Italian Parmigiano, grated (and extra grated cheese for topping at the finish)

1/2 teaspoon garlic powder

10 to 12 fresh basil leaves, chopped finely

2 large fresh organic eggs

Sea salt and freshly ground black pepper, to taste

3/4 to 1 cups water

3 to 6 medium-thin zucchini, washed and sliced into medium-thin slices

Olive oil for frying

Instructions

In a large, deep bowl, combine the flour, grated cheese, garlic powder, chopped basil, and eggs, and season with salt and pepper to taste. If you feel the batter isn't thin enough after adding the eggs, slowly and gradually add water to the batter until it's thick enough to adhere to the slices of zucchini. Mix this well with a fork until well blended, then add the slices of zucchini and gently mix by hand to coat each and every slice.

Let this mixture rest for a moment or two. In the meantime, prepare a large platter with paper towels and set aside.

Add about an inch or so of olive oil to a large, deep, non-stick skillet and place on medium-high heat. Test the oil by dropping a bit of batter in; it should slowly start to cook and begin browning.

Begin adding your zucchini slices and allow to cook and brown until the zucchini begins to soften and the batter is a golden color.

NOTE: Adjust the oil temperature according to the thickness of the zucchini slices. Thicker slices need more time to cook, so don't over brown these — keep the heat a bit lower — while thin slices will cook very, very quickly.

Turn the slices over to cook completely on the other side and then remove them to the large platter and place gently on the paper towels to drain. Sprinkle with additional sea salt at this point, if desired.

Once all the zucchini slices are cooked and drained, remove the oil from the heat and discard properly once cooled.

Serve these at room temperature with a healthy dose of additional grated Parmigiano cheese to taste. Enjoy with wine and toasted breads as an appetizer, or as a side dish to chicken and meat dishes.

Potato, Mushroom & Caramelized Onion Pierogi

Grocery List

Pierogi Dough

2 cups full fat plain or Greek yogurt

1 egg, lightly beaten

1 teaspoon salt

2 1/4 cups flour + more for kneading

Potato, Mushroom & Caramelized Onion Pierogi Filling

2 yellow onions, chopped

1 pound white mushrooms, trimmed and finely diced

3/4 pound potatoes for mashing

4 tablespoons unsalted butter (up to 6 tablespoons)

1 pinch Salt and freshly ground black pepper

1 splash Sour cream or Full-fat or Greek yogurt for serving

Instructions

Pierogi Dough

Beat the yogurt, the egg and the salt together with an electric beater on low until smooth and creamy. Slowly add the flour, beating until smooth. The dough will be very sticky.

Scrape the dough out of the bowl onto a well-floured work surface and knead in enough flour until the dough is smooth and workable (can be rolled out and cut). It will be tacky but not so sticky that it runs all over the work surface and sticks to your hands in a major way.

Wrap the dough in plastic wrap and put it in the refrigerator for 2 hours to firm up.

Potato, Mushroom & Caramelized Onion Pierogi Filling

Chop the onions. Melt 2 tablespoons butter in a large skillet and sauté the onions until caramelized a deep brown, caramelized but not burned. Remove from the skillet and set aside.

In the same skillet, melt another 2 tablespoons of butter and add the chopped mushrooms. Salt and pepper the mushrooms and sauté until they are tender and all the liquid exuded by the mushrooms has evaporated, 5 minutes. Remove from the heat.

While you are cooking the onions and mushrooms, peel and quarter the potato(es) and place in a small pot. Cover with cold water, bring to a boil, then lower heat and simmer until soft and mashable, 15 to 20 minutes. Drain and place in a large mixing bowl.

If you want the filling a bit richer, melt the extra 2 tablespoons of butter and add to the potatoes. Mash and whip the potatoes until smooth and fluffy. Fold in the cooked mushrooms and the caramelized onions until well blended. Salt and pepper again to taste.

Take the dough out of the fridge and work with half at a time. The other half keep in the fridge.

Keeping both your work surface and the surface of the dough well floured, gently roll out the dough to a thickness of about 1/8 inch (1/2 cm), gently lifting it up to flour underneath and turn. Keeping your hands floured also helps.

Using a 3-inch (7 ½ cm) round cookie cutter (they can be made larger if you like) carefully cut out circles, trying not to deform the circles of dough too much, although this dough is easy to work with and "correctable". I lifted up the circles, 2 or 3 at a time, and made sure they were on a floured section of the table before trying to fill and fold. With floured fingertips, I tapped each circle a bit to stretch out the circle. Place a mounded teaspoon of filling just off of the center of each round of dough.

Now, gently pull the wider half over the mound of filling and place the side edge-to-edge with the side with the dough. Nith the edges matching/meeting, just press with the side of your floured index finger, pulling the dough and pressing to seal. The edge should be a bit less than a finger's-width. This will also keep the edge from being too thick. Be very careful not to rip the dough covering the filling.

As you form the pieorgi, 1, 2 or at the most 3 at a time, place them on a floured or lined and floured plate or baking sheet until you are ready to cook.

Bring a pot of water to a boil. Once it is boiling, lower a bit to a healthy simmer and drop in the pieorgi just 6 or 7 at a time (they shouldn't crowd or overlap in the pan). Allow to cook for 6 to 7 minutes. They should float to the top and, when lifted out with a slotted spoon, should look puffy. Cook the rest in batches. Place on towels to drain.

To fry, simply heat olive oil or a mixture of butter and olive oil in a skillet and fry the pierogi for a few minutes per side, in batches, again, not overcrowding. They should be golden

Basil Goat Cheese Toast with Fresh Peaches

Grocery List

3.5 ounces goat cheese

5 sprigs basil

2 slices hearty bread, thickness is up to your preference

1 ripe peach, sliced thick

honey

Instructions

Remove leaves from basil sprigs, stack them and roll them up, and slice as thinly as you can. Mix this basil with your soft goat cheese. I make up a big batch of this and keep it in the fridge all week.

Toast your bread, spread the basil goat cheese thickly (I usually use about half of the amount this recipe makes). Drizzle honey across the top, and layer on the peaches.

Creamy Soup of Hearty Nuts, Apple, Celery Root and Sage

Grocery List

1/2 pound peeled fresh chestnuts (from about 1 pound chestnuts in the shell) or dry-packed bottled or vacuum-sealed peeled chestnuts

3/4 cup Walnuts (Shelled)

2 tablespoons Extra Virgin Olive Oil

1 Medium onion, peeled, trimmed and thinly sliced

1 Medium leek, white part only, thinly sliced, washed and dried

2 McIntosh apples, peeled, cored and cut into 1/2-inch cubes

10 ounces Celery root, peeled and cut into 1/2-inch cubes

4 Sage Leaves rough chopped

1 Sprig Thyme

Pinch Nutmeg

Salt & Pepper

2 quarts Chicken or Vegetable Stock

1/2 cup Heavy Cream

1 teaspoon Tabasco

Walnut Oil, Chopped Walnut and Ciffonade of Sage for garnish

Instructions

Preheat oven at 350°F. In a large saucepan, bring 1 quart water to a boil over high heat. Add the walnuts and boil, uncovered, 1 minute. Drain well.

Spread the walnuts on a cookie sheet lined with aluminum foil. Bake 15 to 20 minutes, or until golden and fragrant. Cool on a rack.

Heat the oil in a stockpot on medium heat. Add the onion, leek, apples, celery root, sage, thyme, nutmeg and salt and pepper to taste and cook, stir occasionally, for about 10 minutes, or until the onions and leeks are soft but not colored. Add the chestnuts, 1/2 cup of the walnuts and chicken stock and bring to the boil. Lower the heat to a simmer and cook for 35 to 40 minutes. Add the heavy cream and tabasco, simmer for 5 to 10 minutes more, then remove from the heat and discard thyme sprig.

Puree the soup until smooth using a blender or a food processor, and working in batches if necessary. For a refined thinner soup pass through a fine-mesh strainer, for heartier soup don't strain, I prefer the latter. You should have about 2 quarts soup. Simmer it over medium heat until slightly thickened. Taste and, if necessary, adjust the seasoning or add more stock/cream to meet your desired consistency. (The soup can be cooled completely and stored in a covered container in the refrigerator for 3 to 4 days or frozen for up to one month. Bring the soup to a boil before serving.)

For service - garnish each bowl with the remaining toasted walnuts (chopped), chiffonade of sage and drizzle of walnut oil

Easiest, Cheesiest Skillet Dip

Grocery List

2 tablespoons unsalted butter

1 large yellow onion, diced

1 teaspoon kosher salt, plus a little more for sprinkling

1 1/2 cups enoki mushrooms (if still attached at bottom when you get them, cut that part off so you have lots of little stems)

1 1/2 cups grated Monterey Jack cheese

1 cup grated cheddar cheese (white or orange is fine)

1 cup grated low-moisture mozzarella

2 tablespoons sour cream, thinned a little with lime juice or water, for drizzling

2 tablespoons spicy honey (I like Mike's Hot Honey)

2 tablespoons very finely chopped chives, plus more if desired

Hearty crackers, tortilla chips, or hunks of crusty bread for serving

Instructions

Heat oven to 475°F.

Set a 10-inch high–heat safe skillet over a medium flame. Add butter. When it has melted, add the onion and salt. Sauté the onion, moving it around only every so often, until it's soft and golden brown and just beginning to caramelize in places, about 5 to 8 minutes. Increase heat to medium-high and add the enoki mushrooms. Sauté another minute or so until they're soft and have shrunk a bit.

Add the grated cheeses, and mix thoroughly with the onion and mushroom. Transfer the skillet to the oven, and bake a few minutes until cheese is bubbling. Turn on the broiler and broil for just a minute or two, until cheese is browned in spots across the top — watch closely to make sure it doesn't burn!

Remove from the oven. Sprinkle a pinch of salt over the cheese. Then, drizzle the top with spicy honey and sour cream. Sprinkle with chopped chives. Serve right from skillet—you may want to wrap the handle with a dish towel!—along with sturdy chips, crackers, or bread.

Artichoke & potato tarte

Grocery List

2 packets frozen artichoke hearts; thawed and drained well

1 small vidalia sweet onion, sliced thinly

2-3 garlic cloves peeled and cut into chunks

homemade chicken stock or vegetable stock (good quality store bought works well but use the unsalted variety)

fresh flat leaf parsley

grated parmigiano cheese

sea salt

black pepper

3 to 4 eggs

approx. 2 to 2 1/2 cups approx. 2 to 2 1/2 cups or more hash brown cut raw potatoes (i prefer to shred my own, but you can also purchase the already shredded variety at your grocer)

1 to 2 oven cooked bacon slices; drained well

Instructions

Using a colander over a large deep bowl, drain and squeeze the excess water from the shredded potatoes and place them in a clean dishrag to dry them well. Once most of the water is removed; add the potatoes to the bowl and season lightly with sea salt and pepper.

Add a healthy amount of grated parmigiano cheese to taste (approx. 1 to 1 1/2 cups to your taste); blend well.

Add a good handful or more of fresh chopped parsley leaves and stalks; crumble the bacon slices and blend everything until well mixed. Using a fork, add one egg to the mixture and very gently mix into the potato mixture until all is soft and the potatoes start to stick together a bit.

Using a pie or quiche plate or metal tin; grease the bottom and sides throughly. Take the potato mixture and add to the pie plate and being to press the mixture into the bottom and sides of the plate to form a crust like base. Try to make the sides as even as possible when pressing, do not leave any gaps in the sides or bottom of the pie plate.

n a preheated oven set to 375 to 400 degrees; set the potato crust mixture in the middle rack of the oven and let bake until very lightly golden brown; approx. 18-20 minutes or so depending on your oven.

While the potato crust is baking; in a medium deep pan, drizzle a healthy amount of olive oil and add the chucks of garlic and slices of onion. Saute on medium high heat until soft and fragrant (do NOT fry); stirring often and watch to not allow the onion and garlic to brown (adjust the heat as needed.)

Once softened; add the drained artichokes to the mixture and mix well; let cook slightly until the artichokes begin to soften. Add a healthy amount of stock about 2 cups or so and set the heat to medium high and let the artichokes cook until the liquids start to reduce a bit and the artichokes are very soft to the bite.

Season the cooked artichokes lightly with sea salt and pepper and remove from the heat. Drain the artichokes through a sieve and retain the left over stock for future use (i love to cook risotto in this left over stock, delicious!)

Once the liquids are well drained add about 2/3 of the artichoke mixture to a large bowl and add a good handful of chopped fresh parsley and a small handful of the grated parmigiano.

Blend this well and once they are completely cooled add in the 2 eggs and mix well until evenly blended.

Now add the artichoke mixture as a filling to the semi-cooked potato crust. Spread the mixture evenly to the edges of the crust; leaving bout 1/2 inch to 1 inch of crust showing. take the remaining artichokes and add a few pieces to the top of the mixture and place inside a preheated 375 degree oven on the middle rack to finish baking.

Bake the tarte until the center begins to firm up and the edges of the potato crust begin to crisp and get very brown. Remove from the oven and allow to come to room temperature and serve immediately with plenty of wine to share and your choice of side dishes

CHAPTER 6
SUMMATION

The cardiopulmonary diet serves as a beacon of hope and healing for individuals navigating the complex terrain of cardiovascular and pulmonary health challenges. Through the careful selection of nourishing foods and mindful dietary practices, individuals can harness the transformative power of nutrition to optimize their well-being and enhance their quality of life.

The insights shared throughout this book underscore the profound impact of dietary choices on cardiopulmonary health outcomes. By embracing a diet rich in fruits, vegetables, whole grains, lean proteins, and healthy fats, individuals can fortify their bodies against the ravages of chronic diseases such as heart disease, diabetes, and respiratory disorders. These nutrient-dense foods not only fuel the body but also serve as potent allies in the fight against inflammation, oxidative stress, and other underlying mechanisms of disease.

Moreover, the cardiopulmonary diet offers a holistic approach to wellness, addressing not only physical health but also mental acuity, emotional well-being, and overall vitality. By stabilizing blood sugar levels, improving cholesterol profiles, and supporting digestive health, this dietary approach empowers individuals to take charge of their health and reclaim their lives with renewed vigor and resilience.

As the journey towards cardiopulmonary health unfolds, it is essential to recognize the invaluable role of healthcare providers and registered dietitians in guiding and supporting individuals along the way. Through collaborative efforts and personalized interventions, individuals can navigate the complexities of dietary management with confidence and clarity, paving the way for sustained health and wellness.

The cardiopulmonary diet represents a beacon of hope and healing, illuminating the path towards a brighter, healthier future for individuals facing cardiopulmonary challenges. By embracing the principles of nutrition, individuals can unlock the full potential of their bodies, fostering resilience, vitality, and well-being for years to come.

www.ingramcontent.com/pod-product-compliance
Lightning Source LLC
Chambersburg PA
CBHW071042240526
45471CB00014B/270